D0951883

Praise for *BARE*

"Susan Hyatt's funny, vibrant spirit has made a difference in many women's lives. Her infectious enthusiasm may be just what you need to learn how to love your body and strip away everything that doesn't serve you."

—Martha Beck, columnist for *O: The Oprah Magazine* and bestselling author of *Finding Your Own North Star* and *Steering by Starlight*

"In some ways, the fact we need Susan's funny, smart, deeply honest book makes me sad. Are we still having this conversation about our thighs?!? But of course we are. I just put on a pair of jeans and automatically looked in the mirror to check how my butt looked. But here's the thing: With books like this one, we are throwing off the stupid and cruel yoke of worrying about our body size and shape one day at a time. We are stopping the madness and eventually it will be a ridiculous idea consigned to history. Susan's book is a bright step in the direction of freedom. You will love her voice, her story, and, most of all, her ideas."

—Jennifer Louden, bestselling author of *The Woman's Comfort Book* and *The Life Organizer*

"*Bare* flips the broken cultural norm—we must starve ourselves to fit into a patriarchal norm of desirability—and focuses instead on strengthening the love, power, and beauty we have inside us. Susan will help you nurture and love the body you are in, choosing health on your terms and in your time."

—Pamela Slim, author of *Body of Work*

"Susan Hyatt is an example of what is possible when you start caring less about how you look to others and more about how you feel toward yourself. Being in your body with love is a skill you can learn—a skill you *should* learn. No matter what anyone thinks about how you look or what you eat, you can claim yourself as worthy exactly as you are. Susan has done that, and she can show you how."

—Brooke Castillo, author of *If I'm So Smart, Why Can't I Lose Weight*

"Susan is the magical fairy godmother/big sister/best friend I always wanted in my life. In *Bare*, she gives me permission to show up and say YES to more pleasure and joy. You'll love this book."

—Denise Duffield-Thomas, author of *Get Rich, Lucky Bitch* and *Chillpreneur*

"Get ready for a beautiful relationship to your body and your life using fierce love as your compass. One of Susan's superpowers is stripping things down until you're standing in raw truth, and *Bare* is no different. The world needs that fully expressed, unapologetic, powerful version of you, so stop hiding and dive into this book."

—Natalie MacNeil, Emmy Award–winning media entrepreneur and creator of SheTakesontheWorld.com

BARE

You don't need a new diet.
You don't need more willpower.
You need a revolution.

BARE

A 7-Week Program to Transform Your Body,
Get More Energy, Feel Amazing, and
Become the Bravest, Most Unstoppable
Version of You

Susan Hyatt

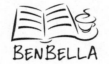

BenBella Books, Inc.
Dallas, TX

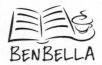

BenBella Books, Inc.
10440 N. Central Expressway, Suite 800
Dallas, TX 75231
www.benbellabooks.com
Send feedback to feedback@benbellabooks.com

Printed in the United States of America
10 9 8 7 6 5 4 3 2 1

Library of Congress Control Number: 2018041822
ISBN 9781946885432 (trade cloth)
ISBN 9781948836173 (electronic)

Editing by Maria Hart
Copyediting by Elizabeth Degenhard
Proofreading by Lisa Story and Cape Cod Compositors, Inc.
Text design by Publishers' Design and Production Services, Inc.
Text composition by Aaron Edmiston
Cover design by Blueline, Holland Colvin
Cover and interior photography by Blueline, Chelsea Sanders
Printed by Lake Book Manufacturing

Distributed to the trade by Two Rivers Distribution, an Ingram brand
www.tworiversdistribution.com

This book is dedicated to every woman who has ever felt uncomfortable in her own skin, not pretty enough, not good enough, or not worthy of attention, respect, or love.

You are worth all of that and so much more.

Contents

Prologue   xi

Introduction   xv

My Story   1

Let's Talk About . . . Dieting   17

Let's Talk About . . . BARE   21

Your Journey Begins Now   35

THE BARE PROCESS

Week 1: Clean Up Your Environment   43

Week 2: Add Pleasure into Your Day   65

Week 3: Eat with Attentiveness   87

Week 4: Exercise with Love   111

Week 5: Declutter Your Closet   137

Week 6: Detox Your Mind   153

Week 7: Show Up and Be Seen   177

BARE Q&A   197

BARE Forever   209

Contents

BARE Daily   225

BARE Careers   227

BARE Research   229

BARE Library   231

Gratitude   235

About the Author   239

Prologue

Her face was tightly drawn. Her body: skeletally thin. Her clothes: designer. Her shoes: worth more than my monthly mortgage. Picture the perfect stereotype of an old-money New Yorker. All that was missing was the teensy poufy lapdog.

I was getting a pedicure at a nail salon, and she was seated in the chair next to mine. We made small talk for a few minutes. She asked me why I was in New York City. I explained I was visiting to lead a seminar for women.

"So, what do you do?" she asked.

"I'm a life coach. I teach women how to stop dieting."

She raised her brows in astonishment. I could see bewilderment in her eyes.

"You teach them how to . . . *stop?*"

I nodded. She looked at me as if I was a three-headed alien from another universe.

"Well, I don't diet," she told me proudly. "I just eat very healthfully. I weigh 100 pounds," she added, although I hadn't inquired. She then went on to tell me exactly what she allows herself to eat (basically: lettuce, air, and steamed fish with no butter or seasoning) and what she doesn't (everything else). *Sounds like a diet to me,* I thought to myself privately.

"I don't get it," she continued, eyeing me incredulously. "If you tell women to stop dieting, what happens? Do they get totally fat?"

I smiled. I've been asked this about a hundred times. And I get it. It's exactly what I used to fear, myself.

"No. Actually, the opposite happens. They lose weight. They learn how to take care of their bodies in a loving, respectful way, and the excess weight melts away."

She nodded, but I could tell she was highly skeptical. I can fully understand.

I used to be the ultimate skeptic.

Ten years ago, if you had told me, "Susan, you are going to stop dieting, and as a result, you are going to lose thirty-five pounds and never gain it back," I would have laughed in your face. But that's exactly what happened.

The 100-pound lady began tapping away on her phone, signaling that our conversation was over. I watched her leave the nail salon. As she disappeared into the manic blur of Manhattan, I sent her a silent, telepathic message of love:

Dear Nail Salon Lady,

You might not believe what I've just told you. You might think I'm nuts.

You might think that carefully tracking your food intake is crucial, otherwise your weight will balloon upward like crazy. That's what the diet books say. That's what the experts on TV say. But I want to let you know . . . it's not true.

As we look back on human history, there's an interesting pattern. Many times—countless times—people have latched onto beliefs that are not true.

Case in point: People used to believe that the earth was flat. Turns out, that's false. People used to believe that women shouldn't be allowed to vote. Again, not true. People used to believe that smoking was good for you. Ha! Definitely not. That's a total lie.

And right now, millions of women believe a different kind of lie. One that's equally harmful. Millions of women believe that something is wrong with their bodies, that their bodies need to be punished and beaten into submission through calorie restriction and grueling exercise. But I want you to know that this isn't true, either.

Millions of women also believe that you have to change your body before you can finally enjoy the life of your dreams. Nope. Incorrect. It's the reverse. You build the life of your dreams—filled with all kinds of experiences that you crave, filled with pleasure, excitement, and joy—and then, as a side effect, your body changes, too.

Just because something is considered "common knowledge" doesn't mean it's true.

The truth might be the exact opposite of everything you've been taught to believe.

Your friend,

Susan

Introduction

We've never met before. But may I take a wild guess about you? I am guessing you opened this book because you are . . . *tired*. So ridiculously tired.

You are tired of . . .

- Rushing out of the shower as quickly as possible because you hate seeing your naked body in the bathroom mirror.
- Avoiding family photos—or ducking into the back row—because you feel heavy and you don't like being photographed. (Being tagged on Facebook is your nightmare.)
- Counting calories, carbs, protein grams, and/or Weight Watchers points, and feeling guilty if you "do it wrong."
- Gazing longingly at your "skinny jeans" and feeling like you'll never be able to fit into them again. (And then viciously berating yourself for "having no willpower" and for "letting yourself go.")
- Snacking when you're not really hungry, or using food to stuff down uncomfortable emotions, and feeling like you don't know how to stop.

- Pinching your "muffin top" or your "arm flab" and feeling discouraged and defeated—like no matter how hard you try, your body never cooperates.
- Postponing important parts of your life until you're thinner—vacations, dating, a wedding, kids, or even career opportunities.
- Feeling intensely preoccupied with food—and your body—all the damn time.

Did I mention a few things that ring true for you?

Are you ready—like, SO READY—to be free of all the drama, all the torture?

Are you ready to stop feeling discouraged, defeated, and exhausted from all the food-body-weight madness?

Are you ready to wake up in the morning, look at your reflection in the mirror, and genuinely like what you see?

Are you ready to enjoy your food—all kinds of food, whatever you feel like having—without any guilt and anxiety, and without feeling that irritating urge to overeat?

Are you ready for more energy, more confidence, more courage that ripples into every part of your day?

Are you ready to feel at home in your body—and at home in your life?

Then you are ready for *Bare.* You've chosen the right book—and I'm so glad that you're here.

My Story

Hi. I'm Susan Hyatt. I'm a master certified life coach. I specialize in helping women transform their lives and their bodies. I've been doing this work for more than eleven years.

Typically, women hire me when there's a painful gap that they can't ignore any longer. A gap between the life they dream about living—and the life they're actually living.

A new client might say to me, "I'm fifty and I still haven't discovered my life purpose. I've spent decades in a career that I don't even like. I don't want to die feeling like I never reached my full potential."

Or "I'm terrified to leave my marriage even though my heart is telling me to go."

Or "I can't believe my body looks the way it does. I'm so heavy. I feel disgusting. I don't understand how I let myself go like this."

My clients range from women in their early twenties to women approaching their seventies. They're moms and CEOs, artists and freelancers, small-town gals and big-city powerhouses. All different types of goals, dreams, and backgrounds. And yet, nearly all of them feel frightened and powerless when we initially meet—like life is "slipping away" and they're not sure how to make a real change.

Many of my clients have tried dozens of different things to change their lives and/or their bodies in the past: therapy, positive affirmations, hypnosis, dieting (Weight Watchers, Jenny Craig, Whole30, Keto, Paleo, intermittent fasting, the Master Cleanse, Atkins, you name it), personal training, or reading every issue of *Shape* magazine ever published.

But nothing has worked, so . . . they arrive in my inbox, inquiring about booking a coaching session, clinging to that last shred of hope that change is still possible.

Good news: It sure as hell is.

I know that changing your body and life is possible, because I've seen it happen for thousands of women who've enrolled in my programs—and because it has happened for me, too.

Before we get into the BARE process, I'd like to share some of my personal story with you. My story might be different from yours, but even if our lives are very different, you may resonate with some of the emotions I share—emotions like guilt, anxiety, frustration, shame, feeling ugly, feeling stressed, or feeling hopeless about the future, like things are never going to change.

Yeah, I've been there. I used to live in a state of body-violence—hating my body, treating my body with absolute disdain, dieting, bingeing, harming myself in so many ways. That was my reality for many years. But today, the violence is in the past. The hatred is over. Today, I treat my body like a friend. My relationship with my body used to feel like a daily battle. Now, there's peace.

I am living proof that this kind of transformation is possible—and please know that I am not "special" in this regard. The type of transformation I experienced is possible for you, too. It's possible for your sister, for your daughter, for your niece, for every woman on Earth. We all have the capacity to shift from body-violence back to body-love.

Here's the story of how it all happened for me.

Pain, Shame, and Weight Gain

It all started with a Weight Watchers pamphlet, a pearl bracelet, and a dream.

OK, maybe not "a dream." More like "panic and despair."

This was fifteen years ago. At that time, I was recovering from a traumatic sexual assault, grieving a miscarriage, and dealing with a tsunami of rage and sadness churning inside.

On top of that, I was working full time—selling residential real estate—and I was constantly overworked and stressed to the max. I was a major overachiever and pushed myself so hard. I slept with my cell phone under my pillow and checked it compulsively, just in case a client needed something at any moment of the day or night. I was a top salesperson in my region, yet I didn't enjoy my work. In fact, I hated it. I felt depressed every Sunday night, knowing I'd have to head into the office the following morning.

In the midst of all this, I was raising my two kids—my daughter, Cora, and my son, Ryan.

I love my kids fiercely. But transitioning into motherhood wasn't easy for me. I didn't enjoy the day-to-day routine of "being a mom" and doing all the typical "mom stuff" that I believed I was supposed to do.

Working full time and then coming home to make dinner, supervise homework, tidy up the house, bake cupcakes from scratch for the school's bake sale, and do the whole bedtime-bath-and-storybook routine . . . it bored and exhausted me. I went through the motions, but I didn't enjoy it. Inside, I was boiling over with resentment, which made me feel like a terrible mom. I often wondered if my family would be better off without me.

To suppress all of the emotions that I didn't want to feel—guilt, anger, resentment—I did what so many of us do: I turned to food for comfort.

Shielding Myself from my Emotions

Eating comforted me—at least temporarily. After a long, soul-paralyzing day at the office, I could zone out with a wheel of Brie cheese, bread, chips, cookies, and a bottle of wine. *Ahhh.* My own private "happy hour" on the couch while the kids wrestled with their homework at the kitchen table. Food was my escape from a career that I loathed. My escape from a life that felt beige and devoid of pleasure. My escape from an ugly, violent world, full of so many disappointments.

I gained thirty-five pounds very quickly. My body no longer felt like my home. I couldn't face myself in the mirror. I avoided photographs and cloaked myself with baggy clothes. The word "disgusting" was a recurring thought. Yet . . . I couldn't stop overeating.

I knew that I needed help. A friend insisted that Weight Watchers would be my salvation. So, I enrolled, got the info packet, started attending meetings, doing the entire rigmarole. I felt optimistic. *Maybe this will really work for me,* I thought. I certainly needed a miracle.

Gaming the System (But Never Winning)

If you're not familiar with Weight Watchers, the premise is that you're allowed to eat a certain number of "points" every day. Each point represents a certain number of calories, basically. If you stick to your allotment of points, then—they assure you—you will lose weight.

Back then, Weight Watchers used to give you a little pearl charm bracelet when you enrolled in the program. Not real pearls, just plastic replicas. Each pearl represented one point. With each point that you eat during your day, you're supposed to move one pearl charm over the other side of the bracelet to keep track. Eat a point, move a pearl. Eat a point, move a pearl. By the end of the day, all of your pearls should be moved over, and when you're out of pearls, then no more food for you. You're done.

Thing is, though, that Weight Watchers has a whole selection of foods that are considered "zero-point" foods—food that you can eat in any amount, as much as you want, and they don't count toward your daily allotment of pearls. Most of these zero-point foods are fruits and vegetables like carrots, celery, and pineapple. Foods that are naturally high in water content (very filling) and relatively low in calories.

The deeper I got into the Weight Watchers program, the more I learned how to cheat the system in amazingly creative ways—figuring out ways to gorge myself without needing to move my pearls. I was truly brilliant at gaming the Weight Watchers system. Like, MENSA-level genius.

For most of the day, I would gorge myself on these supposed zero-point foods. I would stuff myself with a quart of pineapple chunks (no points!) and a bag of baby carrots (no points!) or grapefruit, cherries, cucumber, lima beans, sugar-free candy, or diet soda (no points, baby!).

After carrying on like this, I'd feel bloated and uncomfortable. I wasn't even enjoying anything that I was putting into my mouth. There was no pleasure or satisfaction. It was just a loophole I was exploiting—I wanted to "save up" my precious pearls so that I could binge-eat later without feeling guilty about it. So clever!

With all the time and energy that I spent on figuring out how to maximize my daily allotment of pearls, sweet Jesus, I could have written twelve novels or trained to become a world-class pianist. I shudder to think about how much time I wasted with that nonsense. Time I will never get back.

But back to that pearl bracelet: After saving up my precious pearls for the first half of each day, it was time for my "reward": a gigantic feast at my favorite place, a Mexican restaurant near the real estate office called La Hacienda. My guacamole sanctuary.

I would head down for my midday lunch break—proudly wearing my pearl bracelet with so many pearls to spend—and I would order a platter of enchiladas with gooey cheese, beans, rice, extra chips, and a margarita or three. I deserved it! I had saved up my points for this moment and, damn it, I was going to spend them. Every last one.

I remember one afternoon, after a particularly intense Mexican binge-fest, I made my way back to my desk feeling dizzy and sick. I had tons of paperwork to do and I couldn't focus. I was stuffed, groggy, and pretty tipsy. A coworker stopped by and commented that I'd taken ". . . a really long lunch break." I nodded and prayed she couldn't smell the aftermath of my chip/guac/booze free-for-all seeping out of my pores. I went home early that day because I literally couldn't get anything done. I felt so ashamed.

That night, I remember staring at my pearl bracelet and thinking to myself: *I did everything right. I ate the exact number of points that I was supposed to. So why do I feel like garbage?*

No matter how many Weight Watchers meetings I attended, and no matter how meticulously I tracked my daily points, it felt like nothing was really changing.

I still felt miserable.

I still hated my job.

I still felt an intense urge to overeat.

I still felt angry, sad, and frustrated with myself—and with the world.

Wearing a plastic pearl bracelet did absolutely nothing to resolve those emotional issues. The pearl bracelet was just an alluring distraction—a trinket to occupy my attention so that I didn't have to deal with my actual issues.

This is what a diet is: *a huge distraction.*

I wish I could say, "After that moment, Hallelujah, I saw the light! And I never dieted again!" But, nope. Unfortunately—for me—things got worse before they got better.

The Roller-Coaster Ride Continues

About a month after joining Weight Watchers, I stepped onto the scale and I was elated:

I had lost weight!

Not much, but some.

Enough to make me feel proud and exhilarated, at least for a few days.

But the weight loss never seemed to last. I would lose two pounds; gain them back. Lose three more; gain back four. Lose ten pounds; keep it off for a few weeks; then gain it back yet again. I would yo-yo for months, losing and gaining, dropping out of Weight Watchers and then re-enrolling.

After a year of that insane roller coaster, my body started to revolt.

It started during my morning shower. While sudsing up my shampoo, I noticed chunks of my hair falling out and swirling down the drain. *What the HELL?*

I hopped out of the shower and stared at myself in the steamy bathroom mirror. I looked awful. My skin was blotchy. My complexion was sallow. My hair—the parts of it that weren't falling off my scalp—was brittle. I may have been a few pounds slimmer, but I didn't look "healthy." I looked like a hot mess.

Hair loss was just the beginning. My entire body was in a state of chaos. My periods became heavy and erratic. I felt irritable with my husband and kids. I felt even more exhausted than usual.

My body felt toxic. And it was—because I was feeding myself all kinds of processed crap that was glowingly approved by the head honchos at Weight Watchers. Crap like low-fat processed cookies filled with preservatives; sugar-free yogurt, popsicles, and candies; fake butter spread substitute. Fake food, not real food.

I was in complete denial. I kept telling myself that I was doing everything "right," that I was making "healthy" choices—but looking back, it's no wonder that I looked and felt like a human dumpster. I was filling my body with absolute garbage!

And even on the occasions when I did eat fresh foods— like pineapples and lima beans—I would pack my stomach to the brim, eating way past the point of fullness, and I'd wind up feeling bloated and constipated.

Food is supposed to be a source of pleasure and a source of energy.

But for me, it was neither.

Oh, and the weight that I managed to lose? I'd quickly gain it back. I went in and out of Weight Watchers for years, each time promising myself: *This time, it'll be different.*

Postponing Happiness Until "Someday Later"

Weight Watchers was my first foray into the diet industry— but it wasn't my last. I tried dozens of other diet programs, plans, and systems over the course of about five years.

I lost weight, sometimes, but I always gained it back. It was a continual pattern of disappointment that left me feeling terrible about myself. My self-esteem plummeted.

And that wasn't even the worst part.

The worst part was how dieting became a convenient way to "postpone my life." Over and over, I'd think to myself: *I can't do that now, but I will later. Once I've lost weight.*

Here's an example: While dieting, I didn't allow myself to invest in clothes that I actually liked. I wore clothes that I hated—clothes that didn't fit properly, clothes that didn't reflect my personal style. I rationalized: *I don't deserve new clothes. I need to lose weight first.*

While dieting, I didn't allow myself to take real vacations, to get massages, to have nice things, to feel nice things. I didn't take steps to transition into a new career. I didn't have tough conversations with my husband about the division of labor around the house. I didn't enroll in classes that I was curious about taking. I postponed everything.

Over and over I'd tell myself once I hit that goal weight, my life could begin. Later. Except "later" never arrived.

Hitting Rock Bottom

My little girl was seven years old when she picked up her daddy's camera and secretly snapped a photo of me in a swimsuit.

"Look, mommy!" she said proudly, showing me her work of art.

I looked at the image. I wanted to delete it immediately. It literally made me feel sick.

Despite years of loyal dedication to dozens of different diets, I was still thirty-five pounds over my natural weight. I rarely allowed myself to be photographed—and certainly not in a swimsuit. Seeing how I looked in the photo . . . well, it shocked me. My inner mean-girl went into attack mode: *Lazy slob! You'll never look good again! Cottage cheese ass! Your husband didn't sign up for this . . .*

The barrage of ugly thoughts was almost too much to bear.

That was my rock-bottom moment. I realized that I needed help. Serious help. Obviously, dieting wasn't working, so I needed to find something else. I was willing to try anything. Therapy, life coaching, past-life regression—dude, I was desperate.

I was lucky. I managed to find a woman named Brooke Castillo—a weight-loss specialist who offered coaching over the phone. That worked for me, since she lived multiple time zones away from my hometown in Indiana.

"Please help me to lose weight," I begged Brooke during our first phone call. Before she even had a chance to respond, I broke down crying. Through my tears and snot, words came tumbling out, words that I desperately needed to say. It was a volcanic eruption.

I told Brooke about the sexual assault that I had survived.

I told her about my anger, my grief, and the subsequent spiral into compulsive overeating and weight gain.

I told her how I felt powerless in the face of food—and confused about what I was supposed to be eating and when.

I told her I felt ashamed. Ashamed of myself for gaining weight. Ashamed for not being able to get it off.

"How could I let myself go like this? How could I let this happen?" I asked her.

What she said in response surprised me.

A Radical Choice: Choosing Love

Brooke listened patiently. And then—like the terrific coach that she is—she responded by asking me a very simple question, one that I wasn't expecting. She asked:

"Susan, what would feel like love right now?"

I didn't get it.

Love? Huh?

Brooke went on to explain, "The next time you are feeling stressed, angry, bored, lonely, or full of grief, instead of automatically opening the fridge and searching for a snack, I want you to ask yourself, *What would feel like love right now?*"

Maybe a long walk would feel loving, she explained. Or a bubble bath. Or a great book. Or snuggling with the kids. Or kind words of encouragement from yourself, to yourself. Maybe a nourishing plate of food (if you're truly hungry) would feel loving, rather than inhaling an entire bag of Cool Ranch Doritos.

"Choose love," she encouraged me. "If you keep choosing love, the weight will melt away and it will not come back."

I have to admit, I felt extremely skeptical about this. I had hired Brooke because I was looking for a new kind of meal plan—a program that I could obediently follow. Instead, she was encouraging me to "choose love." Um, excuse me? How is *that* a weight-loss strategy?

But nothing else had been working for me, so despite my skepticism, I gave this whole "love" thing a shot.

When I was deciding what to eat for breakfast in the morning (a bowl of oatmeal with fruit or a processed frozen toaster strudel?), I asked myself, *Susan, what kind of breakfast would feel like love?*

When I was deciding which bed sheets to buy (the nice soft ones or the cheap scratchy ones?), I asked myself, *Susan, which sheets would feel like love?*

When I was feeling stressed and craving a distraction (curling up with a novel or scarfing down a bag of cookies?), I asked myself, *Susan, which choice feels like love?*

To my great astonishment, Brooke's advice worked.

Whenever I paused long enough to ask myself that question—*What feels like love?*—my body's intuition would always point me in the right direction. Every time. Without fail.

Over the course of several months, all of those healthy, loving, self-respecting choices added up. Just as Brooke promised, the extra weight that I was carrying melted away. All of it. Ten years later, I still haven't gained it back.

And it all started with one brilliant question: "What feels like love?"

Choose Love, as Often as You Can

As you get ready to begin the seven-week BARE process, I want you to remember the question that my coach shared with me, and that I've now shared with you:

"What feels like love?"

If you ever reach a point in the BARE process (and trust me, you will) where you don't know the answer to something—you don't know what to eat, you don't know how to resolve a stressful situation, you don't know what to say, what to do, how to deal with an emotion that's coming up for you—ask yourself that question. Listen to your intuition. Follow it. You will be guided exactly where you need to go.

Choose love—as often as you can. This is the foundation of the BARE process. There's a lot more to the process that we're going to discuss in the chapters ahead, but "love" is the guiding principle here, and it's always the right answer to every question.

You'll be amazed by how your body and life both transform—very willingly and quickly—as you move in the direction of love.

Stepping into a Bigger, More Exciting Life

A lot has happened since my first phone call with Brooke, the woman who taught me to choose love, and who helped me to stop the sickening cycle of dieting.

In the ten years that followed . . .

- I quit my job in real estate, shoved my depressing real estate paperwork into boxes, walked out of my office, and never looked back. (About freaking time!)
- I completed my life-coaching certification and then enrolled in a master-level program because I was voraciously hungry to learn as much as I could about the human mind—why we slip into harmful, obsessive patterns so easily; why fear stops us from pursuing things we really want; why we criticize ourselves so harshly; and how we can change.
- I took a huge leap of faith and decided to become my own boss and open my own coaching practice. I purchased a stack of business cards that said: "Susan Hyatt, Certified Life Coach." I slapped together a basic website.

My doors were officially open. (Everyone, including my husband, thought this was pretty insane. "Life coaching? Is that even a real job?" was the refrain I heard over and over.)

- I hustled to line up my very first life-coaching client. And then my second. And third. Slowly—with patience, persistence, and resourcefulness—I took my coaching practice from five figures to six, and from six figures to seven. (Cue my husband's jaw hitting the floor in amazement. He is now a very, very big fan of the life-coaching profession—ha!)

- I studied psychology, nutrition, and the science of weight loss. Lots of people wanted to hire me for weight-loss coaching—especially after learning about my personal transformation—so I studied voraciously, learning as much as I possibly could, applying each new finding to my coaching practice.

- I systematically removed all kinds of toxic beliefs, attitudes, habits, relationships, and time-sucking obligations from my life. My new motto became: *If it makes me feel exhausted and heavy—it's got to go.*

- I started walking. Then running. A mile or so. Then more. After decades of being a couch potato, I reached a point where I felt ready to train for a marathon, which I did.

- I leapt off the side of a sailboat—half naked—and looked at that photo with pride and total amazement. Amazed at what my body could do—have kids, survive assault, run, fly into the future. Amazed at the brave, adventurous woman that I was becoming.

Ten years later . . . here I stand.

I am a master certified life coach. I am a published author. I am a runner. A weight lifter. An athlete. An entrepreneur. I have personally coached more than 1,000 women—in private sessions and in online programs—helping them to transform their bodies and lives through a trademarked process that I call BARE.

So, that's my story. On the surface, it might seem like a story about a busy, working mom who gained—and then lost—thirty-five pounds. And yes, that happened.

But (as I hope I've illustrated), really, it's a story about much more than weight loss. It's a story about a woman who decided to stop treating herself with cruelty and disdain. It's a story about a woman who finally learned how to treat her body like a friend. It's a story about a woman who found the courage to shed things that had been weighing her down—unhealthy relationships, an unsatisfying career, negative thoughts, for starters.

The weight loss? Sure, that happened. But that's not really the point of the story. The physical transformation was just a side effect of the bigger transformation that took place in my life.

Once I chose to stop punishing myself, stop obsessing about my body, and stop distracting myself with pointless diets, that's when my transformation began.

Let's Talk About . . .
Dieting

Dieting Defined

What is a diet?

I define a diet as "Any way of eating that is unpleasurable, unrealistic, or unsustainable for you."

It might be a juice cleanse. It might be a carb-free regime. It might be the Paleo method. It might be a New Year's resolution. It might be a "new life" that you promise yourself you're going to begin ". . . on Monday."

Diets come in all kinds of shapes and packages—and they're not always called "diets."

But if you're eating in a way that feels unpleasurable, unrealistic, or unsustainable, then you, my friend, are on a diet—and diets are incredibly harmful.

Diets harm your physical body. But that's just the beginning. Diets also steal your money, your energy, your confidence, and countless hours of your life. Hours that could be spent doing something else—like spending quality time with your friends and family, writing a novel, hosting a book club, backpacking across Thailand, learning to play the piano, studying a foreign language, taking a seminar to uplevel your career, volunteering for a nonprofit, or starting your own business.

Let's discuss how this destructive pattern plays out for millions of women.

How Diets, Detoxes, and Cleanses Are Stealing Your Life

Dieting steals hours, days, and weeks away from you. Time you will never get back. This theft begins early, when you're just a little girl.

Around age six, according to researchers who study women and body image, you begin to compare yourself to other girls. You begin to wonder if your body is thin enough.

By age ten, it's likely that you've already tried at least one type of diet. It's the beginning of a lifelong battle with your body.

By the time you're a young adult, you're already intensely preoccupied with your body, and you have at least *one strongly negative thought* about your body (*you're too fat; ugh, so ugly*) *every single hour that you are awake.* On it goes, through the decades . . .

By your forty-fifth birthday, statistically speaking, on average, you've tried *sixty-one diets*, plans, programs, detoxes, cleanses, meal plans, regimes, and eating systems in a continual, unending battle to shrink your body and, hopefully, change your life.

By the end of your life, when you tally up all the hours, weeks, and months that you've spent dieting and obsessing over your size, the grand total will be *thirty-one years.*

Yes, you read that correctly: The average woman spends thirty-one years of her life on a diet.

Thirty-one years counting calories. Thirty-one years counting carbs. Thirty-one years counting points.

Thirty-one years spent tracking sugar, obsessing over gluten, weighing four-ounce skinless chicken cutlets, pinching her underarm flab, wishing she was smaller, thinner, tighter, leaner.

Thirty-one years ducking out of photos, standing in the back row of life, avoiding the camera or the spotlight.

Thirty-one years—gone.

It's a horrific waste. Just think of it—thirty-one years of pouring your mental energy into obsessing over your muffin top instead of harnessing your energy to create an amazing life, to build the career of your dreams, to make your mark on the world.

But it doesn't have to be your story. The insanity can stop—right now.

Choosing to STOP DIETING is one of the most empowering things you can do as a human being and as a woman. And the great irony is, when you choose to stop allowing diets to steal your life, that's when you finally lose weight. *Permanently.*

Why the Diet Industry Wants You to Remain Stuck

The diet industry would LOVE for you to keep dieting for the rest of your life. Why? Because when you purchase a new diet system, a diet magazine filled with low-calorie recipes, a slimming powder for your morning smoothie, a book about a detox or a juice cleanse—*Cha-ching!* More cash for the diet industry.

Dieting promises life-altering transformation, happiness, joy, and permanent weight loss—but it rarely (if ever) delivers on that promise. In fact, researchers have found that dieting usually leaves you exactly where you started—except with less money and more frustration.

In the *American Psychologist*, a journal of the American Psychological Association, a UCLA researcher reports: "You can initially lose five to 10 percent of your weight on any number of diets, but then the weight comes back. We found that the majority of people regained all the weight, plus more."

"Diets do not lead to sustained weight loss or health benefits for the majority of people," she adds.

Dieting is like a carnival game that's rigged so that you'll never win. You pay, you try, you lose, and then regain. Over and over. And yet people keep putting down another five-dollar bill, another ten, another twenty, playing the game all over again. *Maybe this time it will work . . .*

Screw that. Spend your hard-earned money on something else. A trip to Japan. A house. A car. A master's degree. A costume for your dog. A philanthropic contribution to a cause that you love. Literally anything else.

From this day forward, you are no longer a customer of the $60 billion diet industry.

You're no longer playing that game.

You're free.

Let's Talk About . . . BARE

What Is the BARE Process, Exactly?

BARE is a trademarked process that I developed and that I've used with my clients over the past ten years. When clients hire me for BARE coaching, I take pride in being the last weight-loss solution they'll ever need.

But let's be clear: BARE is NOT just about weight loss. This is a process that gives you less stress, deeper sleep, more energy, more confidence to pursue your goals and dreams, a better quality of life on every level.

I tell my clients, "If you've got some excess weight that you'd like to shed, BARE will definitely help. But even if you're not interested in losing weight, do the BARE process anyway because there are so many benefits to this process—benefits that go way beyond the surface-level, physical stuff."

In a nutshell, BARE is a seven-week process where you will accomplish the following:

Week 1:   Clean up your environment

Week 2:   Add pleasure into your day

Week 3:   Eat with attentiveness

Week 4:   Exercise with love

Week 5:   Declutter your closet

Week 6:   Detox your mind

Week 7:   Show up and be seen

Each week, you're given a specific assignment to complete. As you complete each assignment, you feel lighter and happier. Your mood changes. Your habits change. Your body changes, too. If you're carrying some excess weight, it melts away. The weight will not come back. Because with BARE, you aren't going on a temporary diet. You are permanently reshaping your mind and your life.

Thousands of Victories . . . and Counting

The women in my BARE programs have sunbathed in bikinis, and they've told me things like, "My stomach hasn't felt the sunshine in over fifteen years."

They've taken dance classes at Beyoncé's rehearsal studio in Manhattan, glistening with sweat, strutting around in heels and twerking to "Partition." (And this was after insisting to me, "I can't dance and I hate exercising.")

They've left depressing cubicle jobs in favor of entrepreneurship, artistry, and freedom.

They've demanded raises, promotions, and better schedules at work, and they've gotten them.

They've come to see themselves as attractive, sexy, and worthy of love.

With BARE, you're not just burning fat and dropping a few dress sizes. You're making a commitment to live your life in a more courageous way so that one day, when you're a beautiful, wise old lady sitting in your rocking chair, you can reflect back on your life and say, "Well, THAT was amazing!" instead of "I wish I'd been a little braver."

What Makes BARE Different from a Diet?

When you diet, you eat in a regimented way to (temporarily) lose weight. You try to stick to the plan. You feel stressed. Your life becomes smaller, more boring, less pleasurable. Eventually you give up. Basically, the whole thing sucks.

With BARE, there's none of that nonsense. As you move through the BARE process, you won't subtract pleasure from your life. You won't downgrade your quality of life. Quite the opposite: You'll add *more* pleasure into your life. You'll *upgrade* your quality of life.

With BARE, you'll take yourself out for gourmet meals and you'll savor every bite, eating slowly, actually tasting and celebrating your food.

You'll declutter your closet and you'll have more fun getting dressed in the morning.

You'll treat yourself to luxurious experiences that you've been putting off for too long.

You'll expand your vision of what's possible for your life and career.

Diets make your life boring. Diets make your life small. BARE does the opposite—**BARE makes your life bigger.**

Why Is the BARE Process Organized into Seven Steps and Seven Weeks?

Because seven is my favorite number! Just kidding.

When I'm teaching BARE, I typically teach the material

over the course of seven weeks. Why? So that you have a full week to learn each concept and apply it to your life.

But feel free to move along at your own pace. If you want to spend more than one week with each step, or less than one week, do your thing! Whatever works for you, rock it.

However, I do recommend that you start with Week 1 and move along in the sequence I've laid out, rather than skipping ahead to Week 4 or 5, for example. The steps appear in a particular order—an order that I've found to be most effective when working with clients.

Also, it's important for me to emphasize that BARE is not a temporary program. You don't "do BARE for seven weeks" and then revert back to your old way of living. The goal is for you to take the concepts that you'll learn in this book and incorporate them into your life—forever. (We'll talk more about this in the chapter called "BARE Forever.")

Questions, Hesitations, and Skepticism That You Might Have

When you pick up a new book—or start contemplating a life-style change—it's pretty common to have a few questions, concerns, and hesitations. Not to mention a healthy dose of skepticism.

Before we dive into the BARE process, I'd like to take a moment to address some of the hesitations that you may already have.

How much weight can I expect to lose while doing the BARE process?

The point of the BARE process is to help you reach your natural weight. I define your "natural weight" as "the weight that your body naturally settles into when you take excellent care of yourself."

My natural weight happens to be around 120 pounds. At my height, 5'3", with my body type, this is a weight that I can maintain effortlessly—just by eating and exercising normally and going about my everyday life. It's not a weight that I have to "fight" to maintain. It's a natural weight for my height, body type, and genetic predisposition. My body feels good at this weight—I have plenty of energy; I feel strong; I feel alive; and I love how I look. That's how I know it's my natural weight.

Your natural weight might be higher or lower than mine, because your body is different than mine. You'll know when you've reached your natural weight because—like me—you'll have plenty of energy, you'll feel strong, and you'll feel alive. Your body will self-regulate and effortlessly maintain that weight. It won't be a constant struggle.

So, if you're wondering, "How much weight can I expect to lose while doing the BARE process?" the answer is, it's completely different for every woman. But I can promise you this:

If you go through the seven-week BARE process—and if you integrate the BARE principles that you've learned into your everyday life—your weight will keep dropping, dropping, dropping, slowly and gradually, week after week, until your body settles at its natural set point. It might take seven weeks to reach your natural weight or it might take seventy weeks. But once you've arrived at that natural weight, you'll know. You'll love how you look and your body will feel "just right."

Should I weigh myself on the scale? Or throw away my scale?

If you currently weigh yourself every single day in an obses-sive manner, then I would gently encourage you to . . . chill the eff out. That type of preoccupation is really harmful.

Try to set the scale aside. Instead of weighing yourself daily, weigh yourself once every two or three weeks to gauge your general progress. But please know: The number on the scale is *not* a complete picture of your progress. The scale is just one of many assessment tools.

In addition to weighing yourself occasionally, you can also check to see how your clothes fit. You can get a body composition scan at your local gym to see if you're losing fat and gaining muscle. You can take a weekly full-body selfie and compare the photos side by side. You can ask yourself questions like, "How am I sleeping lately?" "How does my skin look?" "Do I have more energy?" and most importantly, "How do I feel?"

Combine all of your findings together—weight, clothing fit, body composition, photos, energy levels, emotional state—to get a more accurate picture of how things are going.

I will never forget one client of mine who complained bit-terly that she wasn't losing any weight because the number on the scale wasn't moving. She would moan, "It's not working!" and post irritated messages on Facebook about her "lack of progress." But upon closer assessment, we discovered that she had lost a ton of fat while simultaneously gaining lean muscle. So the number on the scale seemed more or less the same. But her body looked and felt completely different. After realizing this, she was pretty delighted (and felt rather silly for getting obsessed with "the number").

I want to emphasize once again: The scale can be *one* of your assessment tools—but it shouldn't be your *only* tool, and it definitely shouldn't dictate your mood and self-esteem.

In my opinion, the best—and most accurate—way to measure if you're making progress is to check in with how you *feel*. If you're feeling better, then you're on the right path.

But if I stop tracking what I eat, won't I just gain even more weight?

This is a really common fear. I'm happy to share that the answer is "no."

Through the BARE process, you will learn how to tune into your body's hunger signals. You will learn how to eat attentively. You'll quickly discover that your body is really smart. Your body will tell you what it truly wants to eat, and how much, and when. You won't need to count calories (or carbs, or fat grams, or anything else) because your body will tell you when you've had "just the right amount" of food. Your body will become your number-one nutrition guide.

And with BARE, no food is off limits. We don't assign moral values to food. There's no "sinful food" or "naughty food" or "evil food." Good lord. No. This isn't a fire and brimstone church sermon! I don't remember seeing any mention of fudge sundaes on the Ten Commandments, and there's no special place in Hell reserved for Doritos. They're just corn chips, people.

So, throughout this book, you won't see me talking about "good food" and "bad food." However, you will notice me talking about "power food" and "pleasure food."

Power food is packed with nutrients. Power food makes you feel strong, alert, and energized. Think: lean protein, leafy greens, nuts, seeds, fresh produce, whole grains, that type of thing. You know, stuff that is minimally processed.

Pleasure food is not particularly nutritious, but it's decadent and fun! Think: cheesecake, a caramel-infused latte, milk chocolate, French fries, rainbow sprinkles, or a melty grilled cheese sandwich on white bread.

I want you to enjoy power food and pleasure food—both, every day—in whatever proportion feels right for *your body.* I promise: Your body will tell you how much power food it wants, and how much pleasure food it wants, and when.

Before too long, these body signals will become crystal clear, until it's practically like getting a text message from your body saying, "Hey, can I please have a spinach salad for lunch?" or "Please feed me pork chops tonight. Thanks." or "I could totally go for a slice of that blackberry pie! But one slice is perfect; I don't need two."

Again, your body is very smart. Your body has internal signals, checks and balances, and it knows when and what you need to eat. Your job is simply to listen and feed your body accordingly. (We'll talk a lot more about this during Week 3 of the BARE process.)

I don't trust myself around food—especially my favorite foods. If there's no meal plan to follow, won't I just eat like crazy and gain weight? I'm scared.

Right now, you might feel powerless around food. You might feel like you can't be trusted to exist in the same room with a platter of cookies without inhaling at least ten. You might feel like it's impossible to stop eating your favorite foods once you've started.

Maybe you watch other people eating—leaving a cheeseburger unfinished, or enjoying five bites of cake and then calmly pushing the plate away in satisfaction—and you think to yourself, *How is that even POSSIBLE?* It's like watching a Las Vegas magic show. And it feels as impossible as levitating.

That used to be me. I used to repeatedly tell myself that I "couldn't be trusted" around food—especially my favorite foods. (Like seasoned French fries with garlic-mayo dipping sauce. OMG. Once I dove in, that hot, salty basket of deep-fried goodness was MINE. Forget about sharing; you would've had to pry those fries out of my cold, dead claws before I'd give them up.)

But eventually, I realized something:

I feel powerless around food because I'm totally exhausted and bored—and because my day-to-day life isn't very fun, exciting, or pleasurable. Right now, food feels like the only reliable source of pleasure in my life.

When food is the only reliable source of pleasure in your life, then OF COURSE you're going to overeat! Who wouldn't?

I started to seek out forms of pleasure that were non-food-related. I told myself:

I am going to bring more pleasure into my life that isn't food-related and see what happens.

So I did. An afternoon outside in the sunshine with my cat. A pedicure. A long talk with my sister. A cashmere throw blanket and a mug of my favorite tea.

All of those pleasurable activities added up. I felt different. My whole life felt different. Pretty soon, the urge to overeat faded away.

This will happen for you, too. Once you start infusing more pleasure into your daily life, you'll discover that the intense urge to snack and stuff yourself just doesn't "happen" anymore. Because your spirit is being nourished in other ways. Because you're not pleasure-starved anymore.

During Week 2 of this process, we'll talk more about The Pleasure Principle, and you'll experience it for yourself. (I promise you: Pleasure changes lives.)

What if my friends don't like me as much after I change my life and/or lose weight?

When you choose to transform your life—any aspect of your life, whether it's physical, emotional, professional, or financial—two things usually happen:

1. Some people feel inspired. (They think, *You're amazing! I want to go on a similar journey! I want to be just like you!*)
2. Some people feel threatened. (They think, *You're changing. But I'm not. I feel inadequate in your presence because you're highlighting everything I wish I could do that I'm not doing. Now I feel threatened around you.*)

The reality is, some of your friends will probably fall into the first group, and some will fall into the second. You can't control any of this. They're going to feel what they feel, and do what they do, and it's not up to you to change any of it.

My advice: Explain to your friends why you are making these changes and ask for their support. You can say to them: "I am making some changes because I have realized that taking care of myself—mentally and physically—needs to be a top priority. I hope I can count on your support and love."

After saying that, some friends will cheer you on, and others may not. You'll quickly see who your true friends are. It's a blessing to have that information.

I've tried a million things before. Nothing has ever worked. Maybe I just don't have enough willpower to change my body or my life?

This is a very common belief.

You see other women doing amazing things—launching businesses, falling in love with amazing partners, traveling the world, or transforming their bodies—like many of my clients and colleagues do. And you decide, *Whatever she's got that makes it possible for her to do that . . . I just don't have that. I don't have the grit. I don't have the strength. I don't have what it takes.*

Guess what? You are lying to yourself. You do have what it takes.

If you are alive, if your heart is still beating, then you have the power to change any aspect of your life that you want. If you're thinking, *Seriously, Susan, shut up with the personal development B.S. I JUST DON'T HAVE WHAT IT TAKES, OK?* then let me introduce this possibility:

Maybe you have an incredible amount of personal agency and power—the power to shape your life in whatever way you want. But up until now, you haven't been using your power very effectively.

Maybe you've been misdirecting your power. Maybe you've been giving it away—allowing it to be "stolen" or "drained"—instead of harnessing it productively. For example:

Maybe, like one my recent clients, you've given ten years of your life to a career that you don't even like.

Maybe, like, another one of my clients, you spend countless hours each week meticulously planning and preparing diet meals that you don't even enjoy, exhausting yourself in the process.

Maybe, like me fourteen years ago, you repeatedly say yes to family commitments and obligations that bore you.

If that's your pattern, then no wonder you feel powerless! No wonder you feel like you "don't have what it takes" to take care of yourself, or to set goals and achieve them. You're mentally and physically exhausted because you've been giving away your time and energy to people, companies, systems, and commitments that drain your power until it feels like there's nothing left.

But that doesn't have to be your story line forever. *You can change the narrative. You can take back your power—and you can take your life in any direction you want.*

Can you try to believe that? I hope so. Here's a conversation shift that might help:

Instead of saying to yourself, *I want to change my life and body, but I'm pretty sure I don't have what it takes.*

Try saying, *I want to change my life and body. Currently, I am pretty exhausted, which makes the entire prospect feel pretty overwhelming. But that's not going to be my situation forever. Over the next seven weeks, I am going to strip unnecessary B.S. out of my life. I am going to feel lighter, physically and emotionally. I am going to feel my power returning to me—like back when I was a little kid, back when I believed that I could do anything. As the weeks roll by, I am going to feel unstoppable. I'm not there yet, but I'm heading in that direction. Starting right now. I can do this.*

It's time to take back your power—and use it create the life and body that you want.

I don't care about losing weight. I just want to feel healthier and have more energy. Is the BARE process going to help with that?

Hell yes! I have lots of clients who don't particularly care about losing weight. Maybe you'd like to boost your self-esteem, feel sexier, have more energy to chase your kids around the playground, or feel more confident when you're marching into a meeting at work.

BARE is a process that upgrades your physical and mental health on many levels. Weight loss is often a side effect of the process, but it's not the whole story.

I'm a feminist. Is it shallow, vain, or stupid if I want to lose weight or change my body in some way?

I consider myself a fierce, outspoken feminist. I believe that being a feminist comes down to one key word: *choice.*

As a feminist, you get to choose the type of career that you want. You get to choose the sexual partner(s) that you want. You get to choose whether to have kids or not. You get to choose the exact type of lifestyle that you want—and yes, that includes what you choose to eat, how you choose to move your body, and how you choose to express your personality through your hair, shoes, clothes, accessories, and other aspects of your appearance.

You get to choose the type of life that you want—and nobody has the right to tell you "You can't do that" or "That's wrong" or "That's not for you."

Because it's all up to you. That's what being a feminist means to me.

So, if you want to change your lifestyle, change your mindset, shave your head, grow your hair long, get a tattoo, get tattoos removed, change your job, triple your income, train for a marathon, learn Spanish, transform your workspace, transform your waistline—or transform any other part of your life—I say, "YES. Go for it."

Choosing to create the life that you want . . . *that* is the core of feminism. It's not "shallow" or "stupid." It's freaking awesome.

You Don't Have to Do This Alone

When it comes to starting a new process, a new project, or a new chapter in life, some people are lone wolves. Other people like to find a buddy or a community. Whatever works for you, do that.

You can read this book—and do the weekly assignments—with your BFF.

You can start a BARE book club and discuss each chapter with a group of girlfriends.

If you want one-on-one support from a trained professional, you can go online and find a certified BARE coach.

Another option is to join my online community, which is called BARE Daily, where you can chat with women from around the world, get inspired by their victories, and share your own, too. Visit letsgetbare.com (or just google BARE Daily) to find all the info.

You know yourself best. Whatever's going to set you up for the greatest success, go for it. Solo or with a crew, it's going to be a beautiful ride . . .

Your Journey
Begins Now

Imagine that you're standing on a beautiful bridge. Maybe it's painted with rainbow colors, or covered in glitter and gold, or made of strong, sturdy wood with a wonderful scent of pine. This is a moment of celebration, because you're leaving behind your old reality and crossing over into a new way of living. Goodbye, dieting. Goodbye, stress, anxiety, and frustration about your body. Hello to the next chapter.

On the other side of the bridge, imagine a crowd of women. They are smiling, cheering for you, whooping and hollering, and, yes, several are twerking. They're all ages. All body types. Some are tall. Some are petite. Some are curvy. They're waving to you and calling out, "Come on! Cross over! Walk across the bridge! You're going to love it over here!"

These women are my clients. Women who've experienced the BARE process, and who have transformed their lives and bodies.

While writing this book, I reached out to a few of my clients. I asked them to share some words of encouragement with you—a few words to carry you over that bridge, to encourage you to begin this journey right now.

To be clear, these are real women, real clients, and real love notes—for you.

Here's what they said:

Dear sister friend—

It's time. That's why this book is in your hand. It's time to not only make peace with your body but to nourish it with radical loving kindness. Seem impossible? Stick with Susan Hyatt's BARE and you will watch yourself bloom into a body-loving, full-life-living, show-up-for-yourself QUEEN. You've got this. And you have a group of fierce BARE coaches and sisters cheering you on!

—Tracy Carrothers

Congratulations for choosing this book. Choosing this book means you are open to an alternative way and on the precipice of joining a movement to disrupt the diet industry, which robs women of their bold, beautiful life and relationship with our bodies we deserve! As a woman and BARE Certified Coach who wholeheartedly lives and loves the BARE Process, I know you'll be grateful for taking this step. See you on the BARE side!

—Elysa Roberts

The BARE message is one of the most important messages in society today. Period. As a disabled woman—a woman whose body cannot physically match what society says it should look like—I spent a lifetime trying to hide my body, trying to keep everyone else from feeling uncomfortable around me, and attempting to manage my shame around it. BARE has absolutely set me free, and I want to empower every single other woman who has dealt with anything even close to what I have to STOP IT. We are wonderfully made no matter the shape or size. It's time for us to treat ourselves with love and respect.

—Belinda Smith

BARE helped me to wake up and realize that I have the power within to love myself, and I don't need another diet to do that. I learned that it's OK to be big and I can love the skin I am in now. I don't need anyone's acceptance or approval to be the real me. I can stop hiding me and my body. BARE had a huge role in helping me to end my pattern of emotional eating by practicing the mindful eating tools. It's been an amazing ride to freedom. OH . . . and obviously BARE has had a huge influence on how I want to help my clients end emotional eating.

—Amy English

BARE has helped me to fully appreciate myself instead of totally denigrating and hating on myself on a daily basis. I've gained more self-love, appreciation, and confidence. I've learned to love myself. Before, I could hardly stand to look at myself, let alone shine a light and celebrate all my good stuff. It's also connected me to a truly amazing group of women who support, cheerlead, and love each other like nowhere else I have experienced.

—Tamsyn Hawkins

Susan Hyatt is a ROCK STAR when it comes to her BARE program! I would recommend this program to anyone wanting a better outlook on their body and life. And who wouldn't want that??!! Her program isn't just about weight loss; it is about looking at your body through a new perspective and building your confidence muscle. For me personally, BARE has helped me to be really aware of how I eat instead of what I eat, helped me to purge toxic beliefs and other things that don't serve me, like a negative friend or even just a shirt I don't like. What I do know is that my life and my relationship with food and exercise will never be the same now that I have been enlightened by the Susan Goodness! Shaming my body into something it isn't, isn't an option anymore! You'll read this book over and over again!

—Tasha Jackson Hazelton

Through BARE I found freedom from the terrorist-thug-chainsaw-bully that lived in my brain. I understand how she was trying to protect me all along. Now, whenever she shows up I know I'm not showing myself the tenderness that I crave. This alone? MASSIVE! I also learned that pleasure and play is what makes my world go 'round—it's the real fuel or food or nourishment I was seeking.

—Wendy Renee Holthaus

I used to feel unhappy with my body. I felt I didn't deserve to be loved until getting to a certain size. I was not able to lose the weight and had my whole life paused. I was looking for a way to LOVE ME. I KNEW that was the problem but had no idea how to do it. I found myself googling: "How can I love myself?" Until I found BARE! I began to appreciate me and my life, and I lost ALL the extra weight without doing ANY diet, just taking care of my body gently. It felt really like love, not punishment, and I really enjoyed eating healthy and exercising.

I felt it like a big hug to myself. If someone ever told me I was going to be saying this and living like this, I would have laughed out loud saying how impossible and improbable it was. BARE really changed my life. THANK YOU, Susan Hyatt!!

—Margarita Castillo

BARE empowered me to lay down my defenses and start living my life unafraid and unashamed of who I am, what I want, and what I was called to do in this world. It hasn't just changed my life, it has changed the lives of everyone I serve and love every day. Hands down the best decision I ever made.

—Caroline Greene

BARE helped me find my way again after struggling through the first few years of motherhood, a move to a lackluster location, and a career change. I've reconnected with my body and my power as a woman—both things I didn't realize I was even missing.

—Tressa B.

I used to be one of those people who consistently hated on her body. What did she ever do to me? I now appreciate the miracle that is my body, rolls and all. My big strong thighs that have carried me through all of life's trials, now receive daily gratitude instead of hate. I am grateful for Susan's BARE process. It has given me a whole new perspective on what self-love truly is and how living a life of pleasure and purpose can transform anything, including the body.

—Mary Vernal

Girl—put down the little baggie of counted-out almonds paired with grilled chicken and despair. It's time to stop the cycle! Imagine eating what you want, taking selfies with your kids, and infusing your life with pleasure! I'm serious, it can happen—it will happen when you get BARE! When you get real about your body, your desires, and what you really crave, everything changes. No more diets, no more cleanses, no more guilt and shame. I promise when you get BARE, the weight drops, the joy is brought back, and you—yes, you—will fall back in love with yourself and your life. That, my friend, is priceless. So what are you waiting for? You deserve this! The time is now. It's time to get BARE!

—Patti Devin Rantapaa

Turn the page and begin the BARE process. You're going to love how you look and feel. Take a deep breath—here we go. Your journey begins now!

The BARE Process

WEEK 1.   Clean up your environment

WEEK 2.   Add pleasure into your day

WEEK 3.   Eat with attentiveness

WEEK 4.   Exercise with love

WEEK 5.   Declutter your closet

WEEK 6.   Detox your mind

WEEK 7.   Show up and be seen

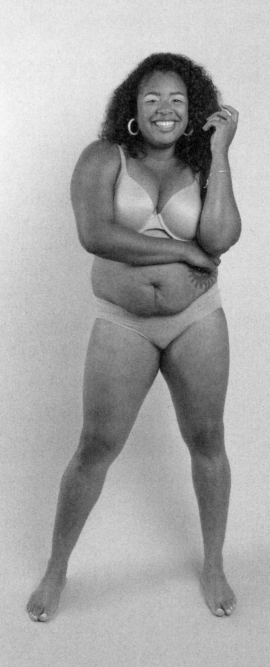

Clean Up Your Environment

Whether you're conscious of it or not,
your environment is shaping you.

Why We're Focusing on Your Environment First—Not Food or Exercise

Week 1 in the BARE process is all about your environment. The stuff that's in your bedroom. The stuff that's in your kitchen. The stuff that's on your computer screen, on your TV, on your bookshelf.

You might be thinking, *Why are we starting here? Shouldn't we be focusing on food and exercise first?*

Here's the thing: Whether you're conscious of it or not, your environment is shaping you. If the first thing you see every morning when you wake up is a cluttered, messy bedroom, that's going to impact your day. If you watch tons of violent TV shows (and have nightmares afterward), that's going to impact your day. If your kitchen is crammed with gadgets that you don't like (and never use), that's going to impact your day.

Everything in your physical environment (your home, your office, your car) and everything in your media environment (the shows you watch, the blogs you read) and everything in your social environment (your friendships, the appointments on your calendar) are influencing your mood in some way.

Your environment might be setting you up for a happy, healthy, positive day. Or, not so much! It's important to investigate and see what's going on.

Upgrading your environment—even just one tiny part of your environment—can make a HUGE difference for your health. Because of this, I always encourage my clients to upgrade their environment first—before attempting to make any other lifestyle changes.

Upgrade Your Environment, Upgrade Your Whole Life

When I say that upgrading your environment can upgrade your whole life, I speak from experience.

For many years, after putting my two kids to bed, my husband and I had an evening routine that went something like this: We'd settle onto the couch with a bowl of Lay's potato chips or some popcorn, snuggle up under a blanket, and watch an episode of *Law & Order: Special Victims Unit.*

If you're not familiar with this particular TV show, allow me to enlighten you: In each episode, there's usually a gruesome rape, murder, or sometimes both. The victim is typically a young woman. You can picture the scene. She's out jogging in the park, ponytail bobbing in the breeze, and then . . . stab, stab, blood everywhere, grisly murder time! The rest of the episode is devoted to tracking down the criminal and bringing him to justice—complete with grim autopsy scenes, dismembered bodies, car chases, shoot-outs, and everything that you might expect from a procedural cop drama. My husband, Scott, loves this show with unbridled passion.

"Come watch with me!" he would plead, almost every night. I would comply, going along with it, not wanting to make a fuss.

But the truth is, this show put me into a state of intense anxiety. Sometimes, after a particularly disturbing episode, I would have trouble falling asleep. Or I'd wake up, panting heavily, sweating from a horrific nightmare.

One night, something shifted in me, and I just couldn't do it anymore.

I told Scott I wasn't willing to watch the show anymore: "You're welcome to watch, honey, but I'm going to read a book in the other room."

Scott was not happy about this. He loved our evening TV snuggle time and he wanted me to be there with him.

"Just read your book in here! You can read while I watch TV."

Nope. Not gonna happen. I held firm. I read my book in the bedroom while he stayed in the den, watching women being chopped apart by psychopaths in creepy basements.

That night, I slept so deeply, and I woke up feeling refreshed.

That was when I realized, *Whoa. That TV show was affecting my sleep so negatively, even more than I thought. That program was totally toxic for me.*

Which got me thinking, *I wonder what else in my environment is toxic for me?*

I started to assess my environment, carefully and attentively, with wide-open eyes. I started with my media environment and then expanded into my physical environment. Everywhere I looked, I noticed things that made me go, *Whoa. Why is THIS here?* There was a LOT to clean up.

Cleaning Up Your Media Environment

Books and magazines

Most of the books on my shelves had titles like *The 30-Day Flab-Blasting Miracle!* or *Drop 10 Pounds in 10 Days!* or *How to Parent a Troubled Child.* Yikes.

In every corner of my home, I was surrounded with books that basically reinforced my worst thoughts: "Your body is gross." "Your child is broken." "You're not a good enough parent."

Resting on my coffee table, I noticed magazines with headlines like "*How This A-List Celebrity Zapped That Baby Weight FAST! Her Belly-Blasting Secrets: INSIDE!!!*"

After reading articles like those, did I feel good about myself? Did I feel empowered? Did I feel inspired? Energized? Nope. It's just more toxicity. It's got to go.

Toxic messages in every room. No wonder I felt exhausted most of the time.

What about you? What does your bookshelf contain right now?

When you pick up your iPad or Kindle and flip through your reading material, what kinds of messages come flying at you, and how do those messages make you feel? Does your book/magazine collection feel empowering and inspiring— or is it time for an upgrade?

Websites, blogs, podcasts

It's not just books and magazines, though. Don't forget about websites, blogs, podcasts, YouTube channels, and the digital places you hang out.

I know a woman who used to "wind down" every evening by reading a celebrity gossip blog—you know, the kind with paparazzi photos and vicious headlines like "Look at Britney's Beach Body Disaster! Flab City, USA!" She would visit this blog automatically—out of habit—and read a few articles. She never felt good doing this. In fact, afterward, she'd usually feel pretty crappy.

One day, she realized, *What the eff I am doing? This isn't OK. This doesn't align with my values and it feels wrong on so many levels.* She decided to stop visiting that gossip site. Cold turkey. She cleared it out of her environment and felt better immediately. She recognized that this site was draining her energy and downgrading her mood. It simply didn't belong in her life. Now she winds down by reading fiction or inspiring memoirs in bed, cuddled next to her dog—a major environmental upgrade.

What about you? Which parts of your digital/media environment boost your mood? Which parts make you feel stronger, happier, and more empowered? And which ones do not?

Social media

I love social media. I primarily use Facebook and Instagram, and I use these platforms to share beautiful moments and inspiring quotes, to share projects I've been working on, promote my business, and chat with friends and clients.

I don't allow hatred in my social media space, nor do I allow cruelty toward women (myself or anybody else), bigotry, or any type of negativity. This is my house, and only cool, kind, compassionate people are invited onto my turf.

If a relative is posting racist nonsense, they get blocked. If someone starts whining about my latest photo, trying to body-shame me ("Whoa, cover up and put some clothes on, Susan!"), they get blocked.

I used to tolerate all kinds of B.S. on social media, but these days I don't.

And you? What's in your social media environment right now? When you log in, do you feel inspired and energized—or exhausted?

Treat your social media world just like it's an extension of your physical space. You might need to do some "tidying up" to create the kind of environment that you want. This might mean un-friending, unfollowing, or blocking certain people, or reducing the amount of time you're spending online to create more balance in your life.

Social media can enhance your quality of life—or diminish it. It's all about how you decide to use it.

TV shows

Like I mentioned earlier, I used to watch *Law & Order: Special Victims Unit* every night with my husband and it gave me horrible nightmares. Totally toxic! But it wasn't the only show. Lots of other TV shows had a similar effect. Anything with intense violence, especially violence toward women, was just not good for me.

I began to choose TV programs much more selectively, and I noticed that I felt calmer and more energized right away.

What about you? Have you gotten into a pattern of watching whatever show(s) your partner, spouse, or roommate wants to watch—even if it stresses you out? Do you feel exhausted afterward? Frightened? Is it impacting your mood? Your self-esteem? Your sleep? If so, it's definitely time to upgrade your TV habits.

From TV to books to websites and social media, there are so many areas that you might want to clean up. And of course, that's just your media environment—it's important to look at your physical environment, too, particularly your home.

Cleaning Up Your Home Environment

Everything in your home is influencing your mood in some way. That treadmill in the corner, covered in dust. That juicer you bought on New Year's Day that never even got unpacked from the box. The nice china that you never allow yourself to use. Every object is telling a story and shaping the way you feel.

Recently, my husband and I were doing some reorganizing in the living room. We've got some older furniture in that room that's comfy but not especially pretty. And then we've got a really nice chair that's high quality and elegant. I've always loved that nice chair. It looks like a chair that a queen might sit in! But it was tucked off in the corner, out of the way, and rarely used.

By positioning the "nice chair" way off in the corner, I was signaling to myself, *In this house, we don't allow ourselves to experience "nice things" on a daily basis. Only occasionally.*

Nope. That's not the kind of message that I want in my environment. So, I decided to put the Queen Chair right in the center of the room, in my favorite spot where I love to read by the fire. I put a beautiful little table next to it with a few books that I love and my favorite teacup.

Right away, the whole environment felt different. It felt like the room was telling a brand-new story: *In this house, we appreciate beautiful things. In this house, it's OK to treat yourself to a lovely, relaxing experience every single day. In this house, every woman is a queen.*

I invite you to look at your entire home with fresh, wide-open, curious eyes. Once you look a little closer, it's fascinating to notice the messages you're receiving from your home. Some of those messages might feel empowering—and some might be due for a change.

Bedroom

It's the first space you see when you wake up. How does it make you feel? Excited to begin the day? Stressed before you even get out of bed?

What do your bed linens signal to you? Do they say, *You don't deserve nice linens touching your skin, just old scratchy ones*? Do they say, *Yasss, queen! You're a woman who deserves beauty and comfort*? There are so many messages that might be coming to you from your bedsheets alone!

Take some time to walk through your bedroom. What is it saying to you?

Closet

Oh, the closet! For many women, the closet is loaded with messages and it can be an emotional landmine. We're going to dedicate an entire week in the BARE process—Week 5—exclusively to your closet, because it's such a big topic.

Bathroom

Does your bathroom environment feel inviting? Soothing? Beautiful? Do you feel inclined to stay a moment? Or does it feel like an icky place that you want to flee immediately, not even glancing at your reflection in the mirror?

Is there a stack of old magazines by the toilet, magazines covered with creepy headlines about "The Worst Beach Bodies" and "Celebrity Fat-Blasting Secrets"? Are there laxatives or diet pills in your bathroom drawers? Hair removal cream that painfully burns your skin—stuff you bought because your ex complained about your scratchy leg stubble that one time?

As you look around your bathroom, you might discover all kinds of things that send a disempowering, negative message to you—things that no longer belong in your space. Good thing your bathroom also has a trash can for taking out the garbage.

Kitchen

When I walk into my kitchen, I want the space to say, *A woman who takes excellent care of herself lives here.* For me, this means having my favorite foods in the fridge, my beloved Instant Pot pressure cooker on the counter, and beautiful metal tins filled with tea. All of these little touches reinforce the following message: *This is the type of woman I am: I love myself. I take care of myself. I don't neglect myself.*

What is your kitchen saying to you?

Car

Maybe you spend several hours each week shuttling the kids to school, commuting to work, and running errands all around town. Your car might feel like a second home!

When you get inside your car, how does the environment make you feel? Do you see spilled cereal everywhere? Is there a secret "nobody must ever know" stash of candy in the glove compartment? Are your teenager's stinky clothes from soccer practice in the backseat, radiating noxious fumes throughout the vehicle? When you buckle yourself in, do you immediately feel stressed even before you pull into reverse and hit the road?

If so, take some time detox your car environment. Invest $25 to get your car professionally vacuumed and washed.

Spritz some calming lavender aromatherapy mist inside. Turn the radio dial to a calming classical music station or preload some inspiring podcasts onto your phone so you can sync it up with your car's Bluetooth system (if you've got one). These little touches make such a difference. It's so worth it.

No car? The same principles apply if you ride the bus, the subway, or the train. Notice how your commute is influencing your mood. Then do something, even if it's very small, to upgrade the experience.

Cleaning Up Your Social Environment

We've discussed your digital/media environment and your home. Now, we're moving into your social environment—friends, frenemies, coworkers, and all the commitments on your calendar, too.

Upgrading your social environment can be tricky because (duh) people aren't inanimate objects like books that can be tossed into the recycling bin. They are human beings, and so things can get a little blurry sometimes. Maybe you've got a cousin who makes you laugh, but she can be needy and exhausting sometimes. Or maybe you've got a coworker who's awesome, but occasionally she makes weird, insensitive comments about people's weight and it bothers you a lot.

I invite you to look at your social environment with curiosity. You don't necessarily need to make any big, sweeping changes today—or this week. Just start to become aware of how certain people (and certain conversations) impact you.

This is an ongoing process, of course. For me, it started when I took a closer look at some of my friendships and realized, *Yikes. This isn't working for me.*

Friends (and frenemies)

Years ago, I was having lunch with a few girlfriends and one of them moaned bitterly, saying, "Why did you guys let me eat dessert?" Then she complained about how fat she was—and vowed to go on a diet "starting Monday." The other women nodded, vowing to start similar diets ASAP.

I used to participate in those types of conversations all the time. But something was changing. I was no longer willing to be part of the "I Hate My Body" Club. It wasn't cute anymore. It just felt poisonous and exhausting.

I became curious about other relationships as well. Relationships with extended family, with neighbors, with parents at my kids' school, with colleagues at work. Some relationships—like my relationship with my best friend, Frances—lifted my spirits and made me feel bold and unstoppable. Some other relationships quite simply did not. I vowed to become more aware of how the various relationships in my life were influencing me. No more sleepwalking. Eyes wide open.

Here's another example of shedding a friend (or rather, a "frenemy") to upgrade my mental and physical health:

About eight years ago, I learned that a woman whom I considered to be a close friend was actually anything but. She was saying mean-spirited, critical, gossipy things about me—behind my back—while pretending to be caring and affectionate to my face.

At first, I tried to talk myself into sweeping things under the rug. I'd reason, *We've known each other so long—and I'm bound to run into her from time to time. So I'll just be civil and polite. There's no need to make a big fuss about this.*

But inside, it was eating me up. Without being totally conscious of it, this frenemy situation was spiking my stress levels and downgrading my quality of life. When I'd bump into her at a friend's potluck dinner, when I'd see her post something on social media, when I'd get an email from her, I felt sick to my stomach. I kept wondering, *Why is she bad-mouthing me behind my back? What kind of friend does that?*

Still, I did nothing. I tried to just put the situation out of my mind.

And then she crossed the line.

I learned that she was griping about what a "bad mother" and "terrible role model" I am. Why? I was proud of my body, and I posted photos of myself lounging in my favorite bikini on Facebook and Instagram. Apparently, in this woman's mind, wearing a bikini—without a huge dose of shame—makes you a "bad mother" and a "terrible role model." Um. Excuse me?

After that incident, I'd had enough. I told this woman that our friendship was over, and that I didn't want to see her or communicate with her anymore. I didn't scream or yell. I was very calm. I just stated the facts: "We're done."

She was stunned. She tried to backpedal and fake apologize. Nope. Not falling for it. I held firm. I haven't spoken to her since.

Without the albatross of this rotten relationship hanging heavily around my neck, I felt a surge of extra creativity and energy. In the year that followed, a series of miraculous things transpired. For starters, I generated more money through my coaching practice than ever before—almost doubling the previous year's sales. I outlined new coaching programs and sold out each one. I had more time and energy to give to my real friends, and those relationships grew even stronger. I trained harder at the gym and loved it. My abs and my booty got more toned than ever before—booyah! Yet another nice side effect of cleaning up my environment.

What about you? Is there someone in your social circle who continually drains you? Someone who's always taking but rarely giving? Someone who leaves you feeling exhausted after every interaction?

You don't necessarily have to end this relationship forever. That might not be realistic. But you can take charge in other ways. You can pledge to spend less time with this person, or only see them in a group setting. Tell this person that topics around food and body are now off limits and change the topic of conversation if things start to feel really negative. You can't "control" other people's behavior, but nevertheless, you are in charge of your environment—which includes your social environment, too.

Commitments and obligations

As I started to examine my calendar, I saw all of the obligations, commitments, social events, PTA meetings, bake sales, carpools, errands, and responsibilities that I had accepted as "just part of my life." It was very illuminating.

Almost every commitment on my calendar made me feel completely exhausted just *thinking* about it. Also, my calendar was so jam-packed there was almost zero time left over for my own health, fitness, or creative pursuits. Not cool.

It was difficult—and required a lot of courage—but gradually, over the course of many weeks and months, I began to subtract exhausting commitments from my calendar.

Goodbye, cupcake baking. Not doing it. (Guess what? I hate baking.)

Goodbye, handmade Christmas decorations. Not doing it. (Why the hell did I ever think that was important?)

Goodbye, afternoon carpool. (I hired a nanny to help

out—and it was worth every cent to get that energy-sucking errand off my plate.)

This process continues to this day. There's always something new to subtract, some new boundary to enforce. There's always room to "lighten up" your calendar and your to-do list a little bit more—and it always feels so good when you do.

Carol's Story
Clearing the Bookshelf,
Creating a New Life

"Carol" (not her real name) hired me for weight-loss coaching. During the first week of our work together, I urged her to examine her environment and search for messages that felt exhausting, disempowering, outdated, and unhelpful.

"Maybe start with your books and magazines," I suggested.

Carol was very resistant to this idea. She explained that she loves saving old issues of health, fitness, and diet-related magazines, like *Shape*, *Self*, and *Women's Fitness*. She never gets rid of them. Ever. In fact, she installed a special bookshelf in her home office to hold her archived issues—ranging back to 1998. Almost eight years' worth of magazines, towering high into the air.

"And, um, why are you saving all of those old magazines?" I inquired.

She explained that she "needs" them because "What if there's a recipe in there that I want to try at some point?" and also because "They've got a lot of great diet plans."

She told me that there was "nothing to remove," not one single magazine needed to go, and, besides, everything was organized very tidily and methodically.

I tried to coax her into the idea of doing a little decluttering. I explained that sometimes we cling to things out of fear, not because we actually want or need them. I told her that keeping a pile of magazines because they include "diet plans" is nonsensical, because diets don't even work.

"You've tried the diets in those magazines, right?" I asked.

"Yes," Carol replied.

"And did ANY of those diets help you to lose weight permanently?"

"No."

"So, you have evidence from your own life that diets don't work. And yet, you're still holding onto hundreds of old magazines filled with diet tips. Why?"

"Well, one day, if I can get more willpower, then maybe those diets could work!"

We ended our phone call locked in a stalemate. Carol was resolute in her conviction. She did NOT want to part with her precious publications, and I decided not to press the issue any further.

I didn't need to. Because a few days later—as if by divine intervention—Carol's bookshelf collapsed under the immense weight of her magazine collection.

At that moment, Carol realized, *OK. Maybe decluttering isn't such a crazy idea after all.*

Carol crouched on the floor of her office, rummaging through the broken bookshelf pieces and the sea of glossy magazines with headlines like "Blast Your Belly Fat in 7 Days!" and "The Supermodel Smoothie Plan" and "5 Fat-Burning Superfoods You Need in Your Life."

For the first time in eight years, she asked herself honestly, *Why am I really holding onto these?*

It was a confrontational moment. Scooping those magazines into her arms, she realized, to her surprise, that she was completely terrified of letting them go.

In her mind, she heard a fearful, timid voice saying, *If you get rid of these magazines, then you'll lose all control. You'll gain even more weight than you already have.*

In some twisted way, these magazines had become a sort of "talisman"—enchanted objects filled with magical diets that, one day, possibly, maybe, hopefully, presumably, could open the portal into the skinny life that Carol dreamed about.

Except it's B.S.—and Carol knew it from her own experience.

The magazines weren't helping her to lose weight or feel happier. They never had. They were just keeping her trapped in a perpetual cycle of yo-yo dieting, achieving temporary success, then backsliding, regaining, and feeling crushed and disappointed.

Carol realized that it was time to officially close that chapter of her life and clear the way for something new. She dumped the magazines into the recycling bin and felt better almost immediately.

During our next phone call, she told me the story of the collapsing bookshelf and we laughed together about it. "An act of God!" Carol told me, and I agreed.

In the months that followed, Carol lost weight steadily and felt a completely new kind of ease within her body. Once she cleared the unnecessary "weight" of those magazines out of her environment, it changed her mood, her behavior, and, by extension, her body. As an added bonus, her furniture wouldn't break apart at random moments. Win-win.

You Don't Have to Change Everything at Once

One thing that clients often say to me is, "Oh no! I am realizing that EVERTHING in my environment is toxic! I am constantly surrounded by messages that exhaust me! I think everything has to go! But then I'll have nothing left! No books, nothing in my house, no social activities, no friends, no spouse!"

To that, I respond, "Take a breath. You don't have to change EVERYTHING about your environment right now. Just change ONE thing. Then see how that feels."

As human beings, many of us get locked into an "all or nothing" mentality.

If you're unhappy at work, you might think: *I need a new job in a new city! Everything must change!* But, in fact, that might not be the ideal solution. Maybe you don't need to uproot your entire life and move to a new city. Maybe you just need to change one thing—like asking your boss if you can tele-commute and work from home every Friday. Maybe that one change would actually give you the balance you crave.

If you're unhappy with your relationship, you might decide: *It's over! I'm not happy. We need to split up. It's time for a huge change!* But hey-o, hold up. Before you make a dras-tic decision, try scheduling a weekly "date night" with your sweetheart so that you can reconnect. Try going on a sexy vacation. Try having a conversation about household chores and responsibilities to come up with a better plan. Try one change. See how that feels. After making one, two, or three relatively small changes, you might see your sweetheart in a new light.

Again, this doesn't have to be an all-or-nothing process. As you're cleaning up your environment, you can take a gradual and patient approach. One thing at a time.

After you've subtracted a few toxic TV shows, magazines, websites, or frenemies from your environment, you might realize . . . that's all you needed to do. No need to uproot everything. Just change a few things and now . . . *whoa*. You feel so much better.

Changes that feel relatively small—like tossing a book into the recycling bin or removing one tedious chore from your weekly to-do list—can reshape your environment in a big way.

Your Assignment
Choose One Aspect of Your Environment and Clean It Up

This week, I want you to choose one aspect of your environment that doesn't feel great—and clean it up.

This can be something really small. It could be one book-shelf. One drawer in your bathroom. One TV show that you watch out of habit (but don't really love). Or perhaps one area of your bedroom.

You could start by looking at your bedside table, for example. What's on that table?

Do you see a diet book (Paleo, Whole30, Atkins) that doesn't belong in your life anymore? Do you see a laptop, iPad, or a pile of work papers that need to be cleared away so that you can get a good night's sleep? Is there a vase with shriveled-up flowers that needs some attention? A bottle of fancy lotion that you never use because you don't treat your body to nice experiences like that? (Hmm. What's THAT all about?)

In one small space—like a bedside table—you might notice a lot of things that you could change or upgrade. Reset that table so that it's telling a positive, empowering, inspiring story to you.

Once you've completed this assignment, write down how it went. Which area of your environment did you choose to clean up? What changes did you make? How did you feel before you started? And how do you feel now?

_____

_____

_____

_____

_____

_____

_____

_____

_____

This week, I'm encouraging you to choose one thing and clean it up. And next week, keep going.

Just like you (hopefully) clean your teeth every night, it's a good idea to continually clean up the messages that are part of your environment.

Every week or so, do a little check-in and ask yourself, "What needs to be cleaned up? What's got to go? How could I create an environment that's even more energizing, inspiring, and beautiful for myself?"

The BARE Truth

If there's one thing I want you to remember at the end of this chapter, it's this:

Whether you're conscious of it or not, your environment is shaping you.

When you upgrade your environment, you're upgrading your whole life, and there's a direct impact on your physical and mental health.

The more that you clean up your environment, the lighter and happier you will feel.

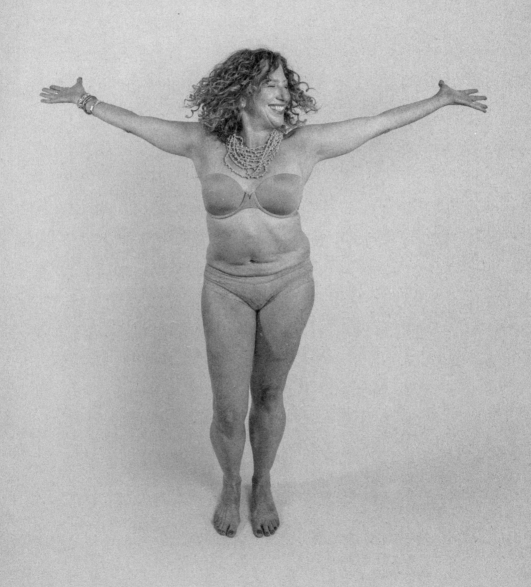

Add Pleasure into Your Day

You're not overeating because you're weak.
You're overeating because you're starving for pleasure.

Why Pleasure (Not Willpower) Is the Secret to Transformation

Fourteen years ago, back when I was constantly trying all kinds of ridiculous diets, I would berate myself for not having enough willpower.

If I had more willpower, then I could buckle down and stick to the plan! I would think to myself. *I'm so lazy. So weak. Why do I always mess up my diet? What is wrong with me?!*

I thought all of my problems stemmed from a lack of willpower. I was wrong.

In fact, most of my issues stemmed from a lack of *pleasure*, not a lack of willpower.

Allow me to explain:

Back in those days, I felt out of control around food. In certain situations, I almost felt *compelled* to overeat—like I was being pulled toward the fridge with a giant magnet, and I couldn't stop myself! I couldn't figure out why this kept happening. It took me a long time to realize, *Oh, I'm not overeating because I'm "weak." I'm overeating because I'm* starving. *Not necessarily for food, but for* pleasure.

So, just as an experiment, I started adding more pleasure into my daily routine: A beautiful walk around the neighborhood. Cuddle time with my cat Moses. Tea with lavender honey in a beautiful blue-and-white china cup. A three-minute Shakira music break. A page-turning romance novel. An inspiring movie. A manicure with my daughter. A moment of total relaxation, sprawled across a soft, cozy throw blanket on my bed.

More pleasure. So many types of pleasure. All day long. More, more, more.

As I infused my life with more pleasure, I felt so much happier, and something incredible happened. That irritating urge to overeat just *disappeared.* It felt like a miracle. The compulsion to stuff myself had haunted me for years and then, it was gone. How? Why? Because I'd been pouring pleasure into my life. Because emotionally and spiritually—finally—*I wasn't starving anymore.*

That's when I realized that *pleasure,* not willpower, is the secret to changing your body and your life.

So, before we talk about what you're eating and how you're exercising, girlfriend, we need to have a big talk about pleasure.

How Pleasurable Experiences Impact Your Brain and Your Body

When you bring more pleasure into your daily routine . . .

- You become happier and way more relaxed. You exhale deeply. Your mind clears. Things that used to be major stressors might not seem quite as daunting.
- Your body releases more *oxytocin*, the "love molecule," which reduces cravings, and which makes you feel sensual, calm, and intimately connected to yourself and others.
- Your body releases more *dopamine* and *serotonin*, two neurotransmitters that give you a positive, optimistic, good-mood vibe, leading to brilliant moments of creativity and improving your problem-solving abilities, too.
- And when you're chilled out and relaxed, breathing deeply, your body releases less *cortisol*, the "stress hormone." With less cortisol in your system, your digestion improves, your metabolism speeds up, and your body stores less fat.

In short: When there's more pleasure in your life, your body can function optimally—the way it's supposed to.

This is called "The Pleasure Principle," and it's been studied by numerous researchers. (Even famed psychoanalyst Sigmund Freud studied the pursuit of pleasure as a driving force in our lives.)

All this may leave you thinking, *Food gives me pleasure, so now I have allowance to eat two dozen frosted mini doughnuts with rainbow sprinkles, because I need more pleasure, right?*

Nope. Gorging on a gut-busting amount of junk food isn't really "pleasurable." Sure, the first one or two mini doughnuts might taste good, but as you continue to eat, and eat, and eat, the experience becomes less pleasurable with every bite. There's a diminishing return on your investment. Eventually, the whole experience is just gross and uncomfortable. That's not "real" pleasure.

Real pleasure makes you feel genuinely happy. It makes you feel grateful to be alive, and grateful to exist in your body—not dying to escape.

Stephanie's Story
How Thirty Minutes of Pleasure Changed Everything

Picture a Hollywood movie with a steely, ambitious, ladder-climbing "boss-lady" character: Stiletto heels. Crisp button-down shirt. Smartphone practically surgically attached to her hand. Leading meetings. Managing teams. Balancing budgets. Making pivotal decisions that directly influence the company's future, not to mention hundreds of people's jobs.

She works around the clock and sleeps with her phone turned on at full volume—you know, just in case there's an "emergency" at the office at 2 AM. She never flinches, sweats, or shows any vulnerability, but you sense that she carries the weight of the world on her shoulders.

That's a perfect description of my client, Stephanie.

When Stephanie hired me for weight-loss coaching, she was carrying about forty extra pounds on her frame. She was ultra-successful and MENSA-level smart, and yet, she couldn't figure out how to shed the weight. She was feeling heavy, tired, and annoyed with herself. She was asking herself, *Why is this ONE THING so hard for me?*

During our very first conversation, it became clear that Stephanie worked . . . a lot. And when I say "a lot," I don't mean quickly checking your email even though it's Saturday. I mean ninety hours a week. Routinely.

Stephanie loved her job, but her "love" was tinged with a bit of regret. She had devoted so much of her life to her profession. She had successfully climbed up the corporate ladder, reaching a salary level about which many people only dream. But in the process, she felt as though she had missed out on true love, marriage, kids, and so many other experiences and opportunities that she wanted.

By the time she came into my life, she had already burned through half a dozen therapists and life coaches. Nearly every one of them said the same thing to her: "Stephanie, consider taking a break. Work less. Play more. Take a vacation. It'll be good for you."

She fired them. Every last one.

"Take a break" was not the advice she wanted to hear. The idea of stepping away from her career, even for just a few days, filled her with an inexplicable level of dread. While she couldn't articulate it at the time, the truth is, without work she felt worthless. It was the linchpin of her entire identity.

During one of my coaching sessions with Stephanie, I shared The Pleasure Principle.

I explained that pleasurable activities and experiences don't just "feel" good, they also impact your body on a physiological level: releasing oxytocin, for example.

"If you bring more pleasure into your daily routine," I explained. "I promise you, your body will be so grateful, and it will be much easier to lose weight."

She was skeptical. She'd been told similar things in the past. She didn't buy it.

I asked her to think of something that might feel pleasurable and fun. Something she could incorporate into her daily routine fairly easily.

Initially she couldn't think of anything that sounded "fun"—what an alien concept!—but eventually, we settled on something that she'd be willing to try. Stephanie loved spending time with her dog. It brought her a huge amount of joy and pleasure. She often regretted the fact that she didn't get to walk her dog in the evening because she was always at the office.

"Starting this week," I told Stephanie, "I have a challenge for you: I want you to leave work thirty minutes earlier than you normally do. I want you to head home and take your dog for a walk. Make this a really pleasurable, fun experience. Your doggy will love it, and it'll be fun for you, too."

Maybe it's because she loves her dog more than almost anything in the world, or maybe it's because she'd reached the end of her rope and was willing try ANYTHING in her quest to lose weight, no matter how silly it seemed. But she agreed to try. "I'll do it. I promise."

She kept her promise. Every day, she slipped out of the office just a tiny bit early, went home, and took her dog for a nice evening stroll. Pretty quickly, this stroll became the highlight of her day—something she really looked forward to doing.

She didn't have to rush. She didn't have to peek at her phone or make any decisions. She just got to walk, breathe, enjoy the fresh air, and hang out with her sweet, fluffy dog.

This feels good, she realized. *I like this.*

One day, she went to the local dog park around sunset. She noticed a handsome guy at the park with his dog. They chatted briefly, and she felt a rush of excitement. He was cute. Like really, really cute. Their dogs got along, too.

The next day, she left work sixty minutes early so that she could head home, shower, and change into a pretty outfit before heading to the dog park. (Hmmm, I wonder why?)

Her evening walks and trips to the dog parks became longer and longer. She looked forward to this nightly ritual, and it became the highlight of her day. Handsome Guy was often there, too, and seeing him was always a nice bonus.

Weeks rolled by. Then months. She noticed the weight melting away steadily and consistently. In time, she dropped forty pounds and reached her ideal/natural weight. She continued her daily dog walk and made lots of other positive lifestyle changes, too. She scheduled a long-overdue vacation. She cut her workload from ninety hours per week down to fifty. She still loved her job and wanted to excel, but not at the expense of her health. Balance was restored. In the midst of all these positive changes, she got a promotion.

The grand finale: One day, after several months of chatting and crushing, she marched up to the Handsome Guy at the dog park and asked him out on a date. He said yes. They've been together ever since.

And it all started with one decision: The decision to bring *just a little more pleasure* into her life.

Like I said, pleasure changes lives.

Honoring What You're Truly Craving

Food can be—and should be—a tremendous source of pleasure. But food shouldn't be the *only* source of pleasure in your life.

If food is the *only* reliable source of pleasure in your life, you'll run into trouble. Common pitfalls include obsessing over food, snacking mindlessly, or binge-eating like I used to. It's vitally important to fill your day with all kinds of pleasure from a variety of sources—not just food. This may sound obvious, yet it's something that so many people forget.

There's a life coach named Rachel Cole whom I deeply respect. Rachel battled an eating disorder for many years. She has written so many heartbreakingly beautiful articles about her journey, and now she uses her personal stories, insights, and coaching skills to help her clients.

One question that Rachel poses to her clients is, *"What are you truly hungry for?"* It's such a simple question—but it's so powerful.

I pose a similar question to my own clients: *"What are you really craving?"*

Initially, you might think, *I'm craving macaroni and cheese!* Maybe that's true, or maybe it's not true. Try to dig one level deeper: "What are you *really* craving?"

You might discover, *Hmm, I'm not actually "hungry" right now, at least not physically. Really, what I'm craving is comfort. That's why mac 'n' cheese sounds so good right now. It sounds really comforting.*

Once you know what you're *really* craving on an emotional/spiritual level, you can find a way to satisfy that craving without turning directly to food.

If you're craving comfort . . .

If you're craving comfort, maybe snuggling under a soft blanket would feel amazing. Or maybe you could reread one of your favorite books from your childhood. Or maybe doing something that doesn't require much mental effort, like folding clean laundry, or organizing your makeup drawer, would give you a feeling of comfort.

A few other options:

Try soaking in a bubble bath or wrapping your hands around a warm cup of tea. Rock yourself in a hammock or rocking chair. Curl up under a ridiculously soft down comforter. (The sheets from Comphy are used in top spas and hotels around the world. UNREAL SOFTNESS.)

Hold a puppy or a kitten—your own or a friend's. Or volunteer at an animal shelter. Don't feel like driving? Visit TheDailyPuppy.com, PuppyWar.com, or KittenWar.com. So much fluffiness!

If you're craving physical touch . . .

Ask a friend for a hug. Or book yourself a massage. If that's too pricey for your budget, find a local massage training school and volunteer to be a practice subject for the masseurs-in-training. Or try giving yourself a self-massage using your favorite lotion or scented oil. Imagine that you're rubbing pure love directly into your calves, forearms, hands, neck, or wherever else you need it.

Ask your significant other to have a sexy date night with you. Or plan a sexy date night by yourself, with yourself, solo style! Either way, enjoy the experience of getting dressed up. Matching bra and panties? Definitely. A silky kimono robe with nothing underneath? Why not! Set the scene. Play your favorite music. Spritz on some perfume. Take a little extra time with your hair and makeup. Whatever rituals make you feel your best, go for it. You can send racy texts to your partner all day long, letting the anticipation build and build. Extra credit: Engage in some self-pleasure before you meet up with your partner. You will be revved up and ready for an amazing night!

(Side note: If you've been feeling sexually "blah" lately, visit kimanami.com for lots of, ahem, inspiring ideas. Kim is a sex and intimacy expert and a vaginal weightlifter. Yes, that's a real thing. And it's just as wild as it sounds. Watch some of Kim's YouTube videos. You will be astonished by what your lady parts can do!)

Or ask your significant other to hold you, spoon, and cuddle. No partner right now? You can go to a *cuddle party*—a safe event where grown-ups snuggle together consensually, fully clothed, in a nonsexual environment. (If you're curious, learn more at cuddleparty.com.)

If you're craving intellectual stimulation . . .

Go online and watch the most popular TED talks ever recorded.

Read a book on any topic that piques your curiosity, no matter how random or peculiar it might be. A book about the mating rituals of parrots? Sure. Go for it. Hit up your local library for thousands of options. You can even read library books on your Kindle!

Get engrossed in a fascinating podcast. There's a great one called Radiolab that I love. You'll learn about how butterflies can see colors that we don't even have words to describe. You'll learn why the number seven is considered lucky. You'll learn why human brains instinctively like to "blame" others. And other marvels, wonders, and factoids that you'll be excited to discuss with your friends ASAP.

If you're over the age of sixty, apply to become a "Senior Scholar." Through the Senior Scholar program, many top universities allow seniors to take college classes for FREE. You're not graded and you don't earn a degree, but you can attend lectures, listen, learn, and study all kinds of fascinating subjects for free.

Under sixty? Check out your local university or college website and see if you can audit a class for free or for a relatively low cost. Check out your local newspaper, too, and see if there are any intriguing talks, book readings, or seminars coming up in your 'hood.

If you're craving a deeper connection with God/spirit/universe . . .

Pray. Say to God, *Hey God. It's me. I need some guidance. I'm feeling stuck regarding _____. Please, will you guide me toward the best possible course of action? Show me what I need to know about _____ today.* Listen for the reply.

Meditate. If sitting in absolute silence sounds awful, try a guided meditation with chill music softly playing in the background. There are hundreds of them available for free on YouTube and in the App Store on your phone.

Wander in nature. Japanese people have a term—*Shinrin-yoku*—which means "forest bathing." Find a local park, hiking trail, or shady grove. Wander with no agenda. Breathe.

If you're craving entertainment, pampering, or straight-up fun . . .

Find a TV show and get REALLY into it! Watch every episode. Google the cast members and read their Wikipedia pages. Watch their interviews. Read their memoirs, too. Give yourself the joy of reveling in a fun obsession, totally geeking out to the max. I definitely recommend *Downton Abbey, Queen Sugar,* and *Outlander,* for starters.

Go to your local salon and get a blowout. Or put a blue streak in your hair. Or if you're commitment-phobic, get a temporary blue extension braided into your hair. (A client of mine did this and she was floating on cloud nine for days.) Or try a wild manicure (dollar signs and gold glitter, maybe?), a face mask, a sugary body scrub, or some other kind of body treatment that sounds fun to you.

Steal your kid's crayons and start coloring.

Book yourself a vacation. Or a staycation. Or an hourcation. Or a bedcation.

Find a live comedy show in your city and go. (Even if it's kinda terrible, it will still be amusing.) Or head to Netflix or YouTube for tons of amazing comedy specials.

Head out for a night of karaoke or dancing, or just dance across your living room.

Try some board games or puzzles.

Google the phrase "dirty knock-knock jokes." Enjoy.

Pleasure Looks Different for Every Woman, So Do It Your Way

Bringing more pleasure into your life means learning about what you crave and learning how to satisfy your own personal cravings—not trying to be just like somebody else.

I learned this lesson the hard way, which also happened to be the awkward, slow, and expensive way.

Shortly after having my second kid, I remember meeting a mom who told me that she never gives her kids store-bought peanut butter.

"No?" I asked. "Why not?"

She informed me that she makes her own homemade peanut butter using a super-fancy food processor. She also makes her own pizza crust. From scratch.

"It's soooo much fun!" she insisted. (And she really meant it.)

I have never enjoyed cooking or baking. And yet, I was awestruck by this mom's elegance, competence, and Grace Kelly–esque beauty. If she insisted that making homemade peanut butter was super fun, then it must be true . . . right?

I went out and bought a big, fancy 14-cup food processor with 115 different blades and attachments. I drove home from the store, filled with visions of homemade peanut butter AND almond butter AND cashew butter AND pesto, tomato sauce, hollandaise, pizza crust, and rosemary-flecked bread dough. *Nigella Lawson—step aside,* I thought. *There's a new domestic goddess in town and her name is Susan "The Cuisinart Queen" Hyatt.*

I got home and unpacked the car. *Time to have some FUN!* I told myself.

But zero fun occurred. I put the food processor in the cupboard and never used it. Not even once. Even just thinking about making homemade pizza dough left me feeling bored and overwhelmed. It just wasn't my version of "fun."

Looking back, the whole thing is pretty hilarious. Slaving over a hot stove in the kitchen brings me zero pleasure, and there are about a billion other things I'd rather be doing with my time. And yet, I thought that purchasing a clunky, expensive food processor would bring so much fun and pleasure into my life! Why? Because another mom told me it would! I imitated her version of fun rather than finding my own. It didn't work.

Maybe you've done this in the past, too. You see a woman who seems to "have it all together" and you think to yourself, *I'll have what she's having.* You try to mimic her behavior, hoping it will transform your body and your life. But that's never how it works. What feels "fun" or "pleasurable" or "nourishing" for her might have a completely different effect on you.

Because you are not her. You are *you*.

Instead of carefully studying your friends, neighbors, heroes—or your favorite celebrities—to try to figure out how to live, how to eat, or how to create a more pleasurable life, turn inward. Tune into your own feelings. Examine your own cravings.

What are *you* truly hungry for?

What are *you* really craving?

What sounds fun and pleasurable to *you*?

Start with those questions. Then come up with a "pleasure plan" that is 100 percent custom-tailored to *you*.

Create Pleasure in Your Life *Now*—Not Later

A common pattern among my clients is a tendency to postpone pleasure until later. Once your inbox is empty, once that big project is done, once you've saved more money, once you've lost more weight, then you'll reward yourself with something pleasurable! Unfortunately, you stay stuck in a pattern of dissatisfaction and stress, always chasing a magical day called "later" that never seems to arrive.

For years, this was my pattern, too. For the first four decades of my life, I dreamed about international travel. London. Paris. Rome. I wanted to see the world. I read travel magazines and dog-eared articles about places I wanted to go. Traveling was my ultimate dream, but I always postponed this dream until later. I told myself I'd go "after the kids are off to college . . ." "after I lose some weight . . ." "once things 'settle down' around here . . ." and a million other excuses.

One day, I finally decided to stop postponing my dreams and just do it.

Once I started traveling, I was hooked. That feeling of unpacking your suitcase in a city filled with beautiful strangers, filled with songs of worship to rituals you never even knew existed, filled with unfamiliar scents and sensations, filled with cobblestone streets leading to candlelit cafes and canals—it's intoxicating and I didn't want to stop.

Over the course of about two years, I visited Italy, France, Spain, and Portugal. Through traveling, I learned that the way I live isn't the only way to live. With each trip, I was continually amazed by how differently Europeans live compared to Americans like me.

Each nation has its own culture and customs, of course, but generally speaking, Europeans don't hover over their phones and computers constantly. They don't answer emails instantaneously. They drive less. They walk everywhere. They take naps. They savor their food, eating slowly, unhurriedly, turning mealtime into a beautiful celebration. They have sex. Lots of sex. Gourmet, high-quality, delicious sex. (One Salon.com article states that 90 percent of men and women rate their sex lives as "very satisfying." In America, it's 48 percent. *Womp womp.*)

Every time I visit, I find myself thinking, *Europeans really know how to LIVE.* It may sound cliché, but it's true. When you slip into the European lifestyle, every day is filled with sensory pleasure and beautiful rituals that elevate ordinary moments into something . . . sublime.

The French have a specific term for it: *joie de vivre* ("the joy of being alive"). For me, *joie de vivre* means finding small ways to infuse pleasure—there's that word again—into my daily life. And not just at mealtime, but all throughout my day.

It means tuning in to my cravings and honoring them.

It means waking up and telling myself: *I'm going to treat myself wonderfully today.*

When I live in this way—with a spirit of *joie de vivre*—I don't feel that intense urge to overeat hanging over me and harassing me. I don't need to turn to excess food for pleasure. My life is already pleasurable enough.

Many people have observed that Europeans are much healthier—and less likely to become overweight or obese—than their American counterparts. *USA Today* released the list of the healthiest countries in the world (with the longest life expectancies) and at the top of the list you see places like Sweden, Austria, Luxembourg, and Switzerland—not the United States. This is partly because Europeans tend to eat higher-quality food in smaller portions than we do. But, I theorize, it's also because Europeans infuse their daily routines with a lot more pleasure than we do.

This is it, sisters. The big revelation that the diet industry doesn't want you to know.

We don't need more willpower. We don't need a rigid meal plan. We don't need grueling boot camp exercise programs. We need to slow down, breathe, and allow ourselves to experience more pleasure.

Not pleasure "later." Not pleasure "one day in the future." Pleasure now. Pleasure today. Pleasure as a regular part of life, woven into our everyday rhythm.

Pleasure changes everything.

Your Assignment
Infuse Your Day with More Pleasure

This week, your assignment is to bring more pleasure into your daily routine. This can look like anything you want. No rules.

What sounds pleasurable to you? What sounds fun, inspiring, and beautiful? Watching the sunrise while sipping your coffee? Snuggling with your cat? Soaking in a bubble bath? Taking an evening walk while listening to your favorite feel-good music? Reading a salacious romance novel? Watching your favorite movie from childhood and reliving some sweet nostalgia? Meeting up with a friend for a long catch-up chat?

Try to come up with one super-pleasurable idea. Write it down.

_____

_____

_____

_____

_____

_____

_____

_____

Tomorrow (or even today, if possible) incorporate this idea into your day.

If you're struggling to come up with something, here are some ideas to help with your brainstorming:

Come up with one way that you could make your morning routine feel a little more pleasurable. Write it down.

_____

_____

_____

_____

_____

_____

_____

Come up with one way that you could make your evening/bedtime routine feel a little more pleasurable. Write it down.

_____

_____

_____

_____

_____

_____

_____

What's one thing that you really want to experience, that sounds really fun, interesting, exciting, or pleasurable to you, but that you keep postponing until "later"? Write it down.

_____

_____

_____

_____

_____

_____

_____

_____

Right now, in this moment, what are you truly hungry for? What are you craving on an emotional/spiritual level?

_____

_____

_____

_____

_____

_____

What's one thing you could do to satisfy that craving? (Ideally, try to come up with something that doesn't involve food.)

_____

_____

_____

_____

_____

_____

_____

_____

Keep searching for new ways to infuse your life with more pleasure. Every cell of your body will say "thank you."

The BARE Truth

If I had to sum up this entire chapter in eleven words, I would say:

The secret to transforming your body is . . . MORE pleasure, not less.

This is a complete mind-set reversal for many women. It certainly was for me.

Pleasure is not optional. As human beings, we need pleasure almost as much as we need oxygen. Without pleasure, we get bored. We feel understimulated. We become stressed and brittle. Our bodies revolt. Often, we end up overeating because we're starving for pleasure.

I passionately believe that if women could get into the habit of being dedicated to our own pleasure, it would radically transform our bodies, our lives, and our relationships, and basically solve 99 percent of our problems.

Pleasure changes lives.

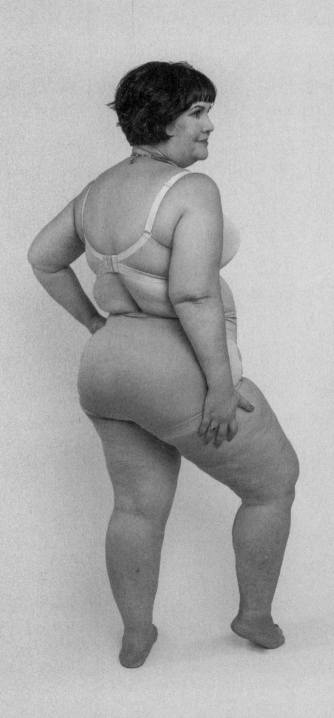

Eat with Attentiveness

You don't need to track everything you eat. You don't need to keep a food diary or obsess over every carb. Just slow down, appreciate your food, and eat attentively. This will transform your body and your quality of life.

What Does It Mean to "Eat with Attentiveness"?

A lot of people think they need to meticulously track everything they eat—either by recording meals in a smartphone app, by writing things down in a food journal, or by measuring food and sticking to specific guidelines, tracking every carb or calorie.

I want to shout from the rooftops, "YOU DO NOT HAVE TO LIVE THIS WAY!"

For most people, this kind of obsessive food-tracking is tiring, distracting, unpleasurable, depressing, and counterproductive. It's like a part-time job—with no pay or benefits!

Instead of tracking, I recommend *eating attentively.*

What does it mean to eat attentively?

It means . . .

- You pay attention to how your body feels. If you're hungry, you eat. If you're starting to feel full, you stop.

- You slow . . . way . . . down. You don't rush through your meals. You take your time, you breathe, you actually taste and enjoy your food. You pay attention to how things taste, how things feel.
- Instead of worrying how much to eat, you tune into your body and your body tells you exactly when you've had enough. When you start feeling those physical signals, telling you, "Hey, I'm getting full," then you stop. (Reading those signals is hard to do when you're rushing through a meal. It's much easier to do when you slow down.)
- Eating attentively also means that you let your body tell you WHAT it wants to eat. You listen to your body's signals. You tune in. Maybe you discover that your body handles gluten just fine, but dairy, not so much. Maybe you discover that one glass of wine with dinner is fine, but two is going to mess up your sleep. You pay attention to how food is interacting with your body.
- Eating attentively also means that you celebrate food! You savor it. You cherish it. You eat like a European, like a French woman—slowly, appreciatively. Meal times become a pleasurable moment in your day.

Some people call this "eating intuitively" or "eating mindfully." I like to use the phrase "eating attentively," "attentive eating," or "eating with attentiveness," because that's exactly what you're doing—paying attention to what you eat and how it tastes and feels.

Children know how to eat attentively. They do it naturally. Have you ever seen a toddler grab a piece of pizza, a bagel, or some fruit or whatever, eat a few bites, and then put it down and head back to their toys? The toddler doesn't feel compelled to finish everything on the plate. The toddler eats until she's full and then she's done! Bye! She moves along to the next activity. So natural. No drama.

But then as we grow older, most of us forget how to eat attentively. It's a skill that we have to relearn.

For me, this relearning process began with a basket of French fries.

Learning to Trust My Body Again

When it comes to French fries, I am ride-or-die. Fries are my all-time favorite food. Krinkle-cut, waffle-cut, shoestring, seasoned or salted, dunked in ketchup or aioli mayo, Michelin-starred or a classic diner—I'll take 'em any way I can get 'em.

Back when I used to compulsively stress-eat to drown out my feelings, French fries were one of my favorite emotional-escape foods. I would scarf down an entire basket by myself, no problemo. Even after the fries had grown cold and gummy, it didn't matter. I'd eat every last one.

Then one night, while out at a restaurant with my family, I decided to try something radical—slowing down and actually savoring my food.

I'd been hearing about this thing that folks were called "mindful eating." It sounded a little hippie-dippy to me. Mindfulness? Really? Am I supposed to meditate about French fries or take my hamburger on a Vision Quest to meet my Spirit Animal? *Come on.*

But then I bought a book called *The Slow Down Diet,* which described mindful eating in terms that made a lot sense to me. The author, Marc David, takes you through a ton of scientific research about nutrition, digestion, and weight loss.

In *The Slow Down Diet,* Marc explains that most people eat very inattentively. You rush through your meal, barely even tasting it. Or you chomp on a sandwich while weaving through cars on the freeway. Or you eat in a highly distracted state—like munching on snacks while hunched over your computer answering emails. You're not really present with your food. You're putting stuff into your mouth, but you're not fully experiencing it. And when you eat inattentively, Marc goes on to explain, it creates a chain reaction of unwanted effects in your body.

For starters, when you eat too quickly, the nerves in your brain don't have adequate time to communicate with the nerves in your gut, which means it's hard to tell when you're hungry and when you're full. Eating inattentively also disrupts your digestion, which, in turn, slows down your metabolism. Eating inattentively can also create a spike in your cortisol levels (aka the "stress hormone"), which slows down your metabolism even more. It also often causes intense sugar cravings later in the day.

Like I said, a whole chain reaction of stuff you seriously don't want.

But conversely, as Marc explains, when you slow down and appreciate each bite, food tastes better, your digestive system can work the way it's supposed to, your metabolism speeds up, and . . . you lose weight faster. Hooray! Upon reading that, I was sold. Or at least—willing to give this whole thing a shot.

I settled into the table with my husband and kids and ordered a basket of seasoned waffle fries. They arrived, crisp and golden-brown, dusted with chili-salt, accompanied by a delicious dipping sauce. I had to practically sit on my hands to avoid grabbing a handful right away. Instead of instantly reaching for a fry, I paused.

I assessed the room. It was nicely lit, relaxed, cozy. My husband and kids looked happy. There was music playing in the background. In the air, I could smell sweetness, salt, smoke, and the rich, umami scent of sizzling steaks and burgers.

I assessed the table. White linen cloth, napkins folded into triangles, beautiful glassware with tinkling ice cubes. A candle. Gleaming silverware. I could tell that someone had worked hard, with great care, to set up a beautiful table for my family and me to enjoy.

I turned my attention to the basket of fries, an assortment of waffley shapes, some large, some smaller, so crisp and enticing. I inhaled their aroma and felt my mouth salivate. I selected a fry that looked especially delicious and I brought it to my lips very slowly.

At this point, I should mention, my family was trying not to burst into laughter. They were thinking, *What kind of demonic force has possessed mom? What is she doing?* But I crunched into the fry—and damn, it was good. I chewed slowly and noticed that the flavors deepened and changed, moving from salty to semi-sweet as the potato starch broke down in my mouth. I ate a few more fries, repeating my slow-motion approach.

Then I noticed something interesting: With each fry that I ate, the intensity of the pleasure decreased. The first fry was epic. The second fry was great. The third fry was good. The fourth fry was delicious, sure, but it wasn't the same kind of flavor explosion I'd experienced with fry number one. The fifth fry was fine, but my palate was changing and it didn't blow my socks off. It was like there was a diminishing return on my investment each time. By the sixth fry, I realized, *Huh. I don't actually want any more fries. I feel satisfied with what I've eaten. I'm good.*

For a moment, this pissed me off. *Six fries and that's it? That's all I get? Noooooooooo!*

I wanted to eat more fries. *All* the fries. Like usual. The part of my brain that was accustomed to binge-eating was seriously annoyed. This seemed like a rotten deal.

But I couldn't deny it. After six waffles fries, I was satisfied. I genuinely did not crave any more fries. Once I had savored my six fries, fully, completely, I was good. End of fry story—for tonight, anyway.

After that experience, I had a small epiphany: When you eat mindfully, slowly, and appreciatively, you don't need as much food to feel satisfied. You can stop before you're totally stuffed—and you don't feel deprived.

It sounds so obvious, spelling it out like that. But I really had to experience it for myself—with that basket of fries—before I believed it.

After that night, I made an effort to slow down and eat attentively as often as possible. Instead of shoveling a scone into my mouth while driving to work, I got out a nice plate, placed the scone on it, and savored it slowly with a spoonful of my favorite jam. *Lovely.*

Instead of mindlessly munching my lunch at my desk, while reading blog articles or reviewing emails, I stood up, walked out, and took fifteen minutes to get lunch at the table—or outside in the sunshine. *Delightful!*

Instead of eating five or six cookies in the afternoon— just because "they were there"—I savored one cookie slowly, appreciatively, and I found that most of the time, one was enough.

Learning how to eat attentively was a huge part of the reason that I was able to lose thirty-five pounds without dieting. It was so liberating to realize that I didn't have to remove any of my favorite foods from my life to lose weight steadily and naturally. I could enjoy my favorite waffle fries, my favorite ice cream, my favorite buttermilk biscuits, creamy salad dressing, crunchy watermelon, avocado, sandwiches, pasta—anything I wanted. Nothing was off limits. I just had to eat a bit slower, and, in certain instances, a bit less.

Learning how to eat attentively changed my body—and changed my whole life.

Your body desperately wants you to slow down—and it will respond appreciatively when you do. You'll lose weight, and it won't feel like hard work, because eating will actually bring more pleasure, not less.

How to Figure Out When It's Time to Stop Eating

When I talk about eating attentively, my clients have a lot of questions, including:

- How can I tell when I should eat something?
- How can I tell when I have eaten just the right amount?
- How can I tell when I have eaten too much?

There's a great system for this called "the hunger scale." Here's how it works: Picture a scale going from –5 to 5.

Each number of the scale represents a level of hunger or fullness:

–5. I am so hungry, I could eat this table, the tablecloth, my fork, my beloved child, anything. I am starving. The room is spinning. I am going berserk with hunger.

–4. I am so hungry, I would eat just about anything placed in front of me, even food that I don't particularly like. Anything will do. Seriously. I need food ASAP.

–3. I am really hungry. My stomach is growling loudly. I feel weak and lightheaded. Maybe a little cranky.

BARE Hunger Scale

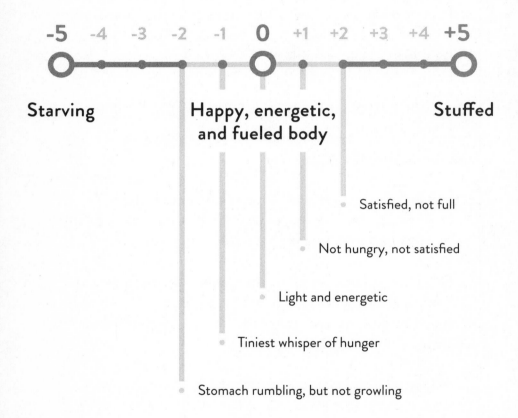

-5   -4   -3   -2   -1   0   +1   +2   +3   +4   +5

Starving

Happy, energetic,
and fueled body

Stuffed

Satisfied, not full

Not hungry, not satisfied

Light and energetic

Tiniest whisper of hunger

Stomach rumbling, but not growling

Borrowed from the remarkable work of Brooke Castillo.

−2. I am hungry. I don't feel weak and lightheaded yet, but it's definitely time to eat something.

−1. I am not super hungry yet, but I am getting there. It's probably time to start figuring out when/where I'm going to have my next meal.

0. I am not super hungry. I am not super full. I feel neutral. (I probably had a meal or a snack within the last hour or so.)

+1. I've had some food and I feel fairly satisfied. I could probably eat a bit more, but I don't necessarily have to.

+2. I am satisfied. Not stuffed. Just right. This would be a good time to stop eating before I get too full.

+3. I am too full. Not super-gross full, but I definitely overdid it a bit. I'm sleepy.

+4. I overate quite a bit. Way too full. I feel like I'm going to slip into a food coma.

+5. I am in pain. My stomach feels so full; it's really uncomfortable. I need to lie down in a dark room, and I don't want anyone around me. This sucks.

The best way to eat is to stay between −2 and +2. You don't want to allow yourself to get too hungry or too full. The aim is to keep your body in that middle zone.

If you've allowed yourself to reach −3 hunger, then you're way too hungry. You're more likely to make poor food choices, and you're more likely to overeat at your next meal because your body is panicking. Also, when your body thinks you are starving, it cues your metabolism to slow down to preserve energy. So, reaching −3, −4, or −5 hunger is a bad idea for a variety of reasons.

Conversely, if you've allowed yourself to reach +3 fullness, then you're too full, and you probably feel sleepy and uncomfortable. Your digestive system has to work extra-hard to process all the excess food. The rest of your day won't be particularly productive. If you reach **+3, +4,** or **+5** on a regular basis, that means you're consistently overfeeding your body, and you'll gain weight.

Here's the good news: When you slow down and eat attentively, it becomes a lot easier to check in with your body to determine your level of hunger. On the flip side, when you rush through your meal, it's a lot harder to tell. When you are fully present with your meal, you're giving your body a chance to communicate with you—and let you know where you are on the hunger scale.

Your New Food Philosophy: Nothing Is Off Limits

Back when I was bouncing from diet to diet—Weight Watchers, Atkins, South Beach—I put food into two categories:

1. Food that makes me skinny
2. Food that makes me fat

I didn't care if a particular food was nutritious or delicious or packed with chemicals. If I thought a particular food would make me skinny, I would eat it. And of course, it all depended on which diet plan I was loyally following at the moment.

While I was doing Atkins, I was told that bacon is a food that would make me skinny. Then my life became a festival of crispy bacon, eggs, cheese, and other foods that are approved by the Atkins system. I'd eat bacon until bacon grease was practically seeping out of my pores. I'd eat bacon until I was actually sick of the sight of bacon. (Which, believe me, is no easy feat for a bacon lover like me.)

While I was doing Weight Watchers, I was told that low-calorie frozen desserts are a great choice. Excellent! Only one point per treat! These desserts have an ingredient list that's so long and convoluted, it's basically unpronounceable. They're laden with so many preservatives, they'll probably outlive me and my entire family. No matter! I would eat several of them in one sitting because, supposedly, they'll make me skinny.

I felt proud of myself for eating "skinny food." I felt guilty for eating "fat food." So many emotions, twisted up into each meal. Not surprisingly, very few meals felt genuinely satisfying. I always left the table feeling hungry—physically hungry, or emotionally and spiritually hungry. While dieting, I always felt deprived.

I hear the same story line from so many of my clients. I hear my clients talk about:

- Good food and bad food
- Guilt-free food and evil food
- Healthy food and sinful food

Here's a wild notion: What if food isn't "good" or "evil"? What if food is just . . . food?

What if you're allowed to eat whatever types of food you want, every single day, in whatever amount feels right for your body?

What if nothing is off limits?

And what if you could lose weight—and keep it off permanently—by doing this?

When I introduce these wild notions to my clients, most of them respond by saying, "Nuh uh, no way! That won't work for me."

Then they tell me, "No, you don't understand. When I start eating food that I really love—like ice cream—I literally can't stop."

"Maybe other people can eat whatever they want and 'stop' at a certain point, before they're too full," they say. "But not me. I can't be trusted around food like that. I'm the kind of person who needs some type of structured plan to follow. Can you give me a meal plan?"

I understand the desire for structure, for some type of plan. Just like most of my clients, I used to believe that I couldn't be trusted to be in the same room as a platter of gooey fudge brownies without inhaling every last crumb and licking the pan clean. Ten years ago, I probably would have done exactly that.

But I now know that it is absolutely possible to have one brownie, or six French fries, or five bites of carrot cake . . . savor each bite, feel satisfied, and stop there.

It might seem inconceivable right now. You might not believe me. You might think I don't understand what it's like for you, that I don't understand the intense urges you feel, that I don't understand the lack of willpower that you have.

I do understand. I've been there, staring into the bottom of an empty supersize bag of Lay's chips and feeling like an absolute garbage heap of a human being. I know what that pain feels like.

I am telling you—as a woman who has crossed over to the other side of the rainbow—that *it is possible* to change your relationship with food, and *it is possible* to transform your body and your life.

But to do that, you've got to be willing to stop labeling food as "good" and "evil," you've got to be willing to eat more attentively, and you've got to be willing to stop depriving and punishing yourself. In other words: you've got to be willing to stop dieting.

Because when you're dieting, or following any type of prescribed meal plan, you're allowing an external system/program/guru to tell you what to eat and how much and when, instead of relying on your body's natural signals of hunger and fullness. You're putting the power of when and how to feed yourself in the hands of an outside source instead of trusting your own body's wisdom.

But when you take back your personal power and start trusting and listening to your body, that's when things finally start to change.

Power Food and Pleasure Food

I no longer put food into good/bad categories. Instead, as I've mentioned, I think about food in terms of *power* and *pleasure.* Here's a little more on how I define them . . .

Power food makes you feel strong and energized. Fruit. Veggies. Nuts. Lean protein. Whole grains. High-quality dairy. Healthy fats, like olive oil, coconut oil, or a dollop of organic butter. Power food is nutritious and leaves you feeling "powered up" rather than sluggish. Power food is stuff that's made fresh. Stuff that's minimally processed. Stuff that doesn't come out of a frozen food box or a plastic sleeve. Real, actual food that's full of vitamins, minerals, and all the nutrients that your body needs to function at its best.

Pleasure food is not particularly nutritious, but it's decadent and fun! Pleasure food includes alcoholic beverages, candy, cake, cookies, pastries, soda pop, milkshakes, chips, French fries—basically, any food that's purely just for pleasure.

A smoothie that's packed with kale, pineapple, coconut

milk, almond butter, and flax and chia seeds would be considered power food. A root beer float with vanilla ice cream? That's pleasure food. A grilled chicken wrap with sprouts, avocado, and roasted tomatoes tucked inside a whole grain tortilla? Power food. A flaky croissant filled with bacon and melted cheese? Pleasure food. You get the idea. This is common sense stuff.

If you *only* eat power food, you're probably going to feel deprived, irritable, and annoyed, and you'll have obsessive thoughts about all the pleasure food that you love but aren't getting. (The more you refuse to let yourself have some pleasure food, the more you'll want it!)

If you *only* eat pleasure food, you're probably going to feel lethargic, foggy, and bloated, and you might develop health issues due to nutritional deficiencies.

The goal is to find a happy balance of power food and pleasure food. Enjoy both!

Women always want to know, "But how much power food? And how much pleasure food? Is there a particular ratio or proportion that I ought to be following? What should I dooo-ooo?"

In response to these questions, I always tell my clients, "Don't worry about adhering to a specific ratio. And don't worry about what the woman sitting next to you is eating. She's not you. Everyone's body is different. Just relax, eat attentively, and notice how your body feels after each meal. Enjoy power food and pleasure food every day . . . in whatever proportion feels good for *your* body."

The proportion of power/pleasure food that "feels good" may change from day to day, and from year to year. What feels right for your body at age forty-five might be different from what feels right at twenty-five, or sixty-five, or when you're pregnant, breastfeeding, or recovering from an illness.

Always tune in to your body and notice how you feel during and after meals. Your body will tell you what it needs.

The bottom line is . . . when you enjoy power food and pleasure food (*both*, not just one or the other), it feels physically and emotionally satisfying. It feels awesome. It feels sustainable. You feel like, "I'm getting everything I need and want. I don't feel deprived. I feel great!"

Yes, It Does Get Easier

After a lifetime of eating quickly and inattentively, you may find it hard to slow down. Likewise, if you're used to pushing your body into a state of being starving or totally stuffed, eating attentively might feel strange at first. It can feel emotional. Intense. You might find yourself sitting there, trying to savor each bite appreciatively, but inside, you're secretly thinking, *This sucks. I just want to eat the ENTIRE pint of ice cream! Ugh. When will that urge go away? Will it always be this hard?*

No, it will not always be this hard.

Eating attentively becomes easier the more that you practice. It really does. Eventually, you'll be a total pro. Mealtime will be a completely different experience.

Case in point: About a month ago, I went out for dinner at my favorite local restaurant. They had a gigantic carrot cake on the counter. It had buttercream frosting. My absolute favorite. I asked the waiter if it was fresh. Oh yes. So fresh. It had been baked earlier that day. My mouth started watering, and I ordered a slice to share with my husband.

They brought us a massive slice of cake. It was the size of a small child. I took the first bite and I was so glad I ordered it. So many places make buttercream frosting too stiff, or too sweet, but this—this was perfection. I took a second bite. Then a third, fourth, and fifth. After the fifth bite, I set down my fork and I realized, *That was delicious, but I think I'm done. I can stop right there.*

It wasn't a battle. It wasn't a challenge. I didn't have to wrestle with my emotions and pound myself into submission. I didn't have to beg the waiter to take it out of my sight. I just . . . stopped eating the cake. It was that easy.

Eleven years ago, I didn't think it was humanly possible to do something like that. But now? I've reached a point where eating attentively is so natural and so effortless, I barely even have to think about it. My body tells me when it's had enough food. And I stop eating. The end. That's it. No big drama.

It feels like magic. After all, this is coming from a woman who used to inhale entire trays of French fries dunked in mayonnaise—and who used to gorge on pineapple chunks (and other "zero point" Weight Watchers foods) until I was so full, I wanted to cry.

Thanks to being present with my food, I completely transformed my relationship with it. I got to a point where I can have five bites of the most decadent cake on planet Earth, love each bite, and stop there, feeling genuinely satisfied.

I promise, you can get to that point, too. It all starts when you slow yourself down—and start treating your food with more respect and appreciation. Your body will say "thank you" in so many ways.

Callie's Story
The Power of a Cloth Napkin

Have you ever cried happy tears because of a napkin-related story? I have.

As a Southern woman, born and raised in Savannah, Georgia, I've always been very fond of fancy linen napkins—the kind that your auntie or grandma might bring out for a special Sunday supper.

To me, cloth napkins have always represented love and celebration. Seeing a cloth napkin immediately brings me back to my childhood and sends the signal: This is a special moment. Celebrate. Enjoy it. Savor it.

During my kitchen remodel, I asked the contractor to install a special napkin drawer where I could organize and display my collection of fancy napkins. There's one with a fox—in honor of my husband Scott, aka the Silver Fox. There's one with a sailboat. There's a monogrammed set with our initials. And on and on and on it goes. (Life goal: to become a highly eccentric elderly lady with hundreds of incredible napkins, and an equal number of shoes, all worthy of being displayed at the Owens-Thomas House museum in Savannah. I'm well on my way to achieving that goal!)

Once the napkin drawer was complete, it brought me an unreasonable amount of joy. I kept opening it and closing it, marveling in delight. All those pretty napkins, lined up so neatly!

Obviously, I had to take a photo to share with my friends and clients on Facebook. "I love these napkins because they make mealtime feel extra beautiful. These napkins inspire me to slow down and really savor my food. It makes the whole experience so much better," I explained in the post.

That photo sparked a lively little discussion. Lots of women agreed: Yes, slowing down feels so good, and yes, cloth napkins are an undercelebrated treasure! Out with paper nonsense! Bring back the linens!

One woman—a new client of mine named Callie—felt so excited by the photo that she went out and bought her very own set of fancy cloth napkins. She emailed me later to show me a photo. I squealed with excitement when I saw it, and we shared a moment of mutual napkin appreciation.

Callie has five kids and, as you might imagine, her daily life is a swirl of unending chores, cleaning, and general chaos. Mealtime is especially chaotic. Typically, her kids will crowd around the table, fighting over the last hot dog, while Callie washes dishes in the background. She rarely sits down at the table—often, she'll pick uneaten pieces of food off her kids' plates or spoon leftover macaroni directly from the pan into her mouth. Not exactly a Michelin-starred experience.

After hiring me for weight-loss coaching, Callie decided to start a new evening ritual. After feeding the kids and getting them off to bed, she would take out one of her new cloth napkins—so crisp and freshly pressed—and she'd sit down at the table for a peaceful, quiet dinner, either alone or with her husband.

The cloth napkin became a symbol for all of the feelings that Callie was desperately craving: peace, quiet, calm, civility, and dignity. Every time she laid it out on the table, it was like a visual trigger, reminding her to slow down and take a moment for herself. She started carrying a cloth napkin with her every-where—even on airplanes.

"Every time I see that napkin," Callie told me, "It's like a reminder that 'I deserve nice things and nice experiences' and that 'I matter, too.'"

To date, Callie has lost forty-five pounds. She still wrangles a huge amount of responsibility every day. But her relationship with food, and with her body, has completely changed. Instead of hunching over the sink shoveling cold, gummy pasta into her mouth at the end of a long, stressful day, she pulls out her cloth napkin and creates a nourishing dinner experience for herself. It's a small ritual, yet the implications are huge. It's a moment of peace and sensory pleasure that was sorely lacking in Callie's life, and that she has chosen to restore.

The napkin has become a symbol of respect—the respect that Callie deserves.

You *Really* Don't Need to Count Carbs or Calories

So many women have said to me, "But Susan, you don't understand; I'm the sort of person who just NEEDS to track calories/points/carbs/etc. I need structure. I need accountability. Otherwise everything spirals out of control. Eating attentively sounds nice in theory, but I know it won't work for me."

Uh huh. I hear you, and . . . I respectfully disagree. Consider this:

You can pay attention to your finances . . . without obsessing about your money and checking your bank account balance every ten minutes and tracking each dime like a hawk.

You can pay attention to your kids . . . without obsessing about your children and texting the babysitter every five seconds to make sure they're OK.

Similarly, you can pay attention to your food . . . without constantly thinking about your food and obsessively tracking every morsel, every gram of fat, every carb and calorie.

It's all about balance. Finding a middle ground. Not ignoring food, but not obsessing about it, either. My wish for you—and for every woman—is to shift from obsessing to simply paying attention. You can start with your very next meal.

Your Assignment
Take Yourself Out for a Beautiful Meal

This week, your assignment is to experience what it feels like to eat attentively by taking yourself out for a meal at a restaurant that you love.

Try to resist bringing along your phone, tablet, or Kindle. Make this a special, screen-free meal experience. If you'd like to bring along a notebook and pen to record your thoughts and feelings throughout your meal, that's fine.

As you settle into your table, notice your surroundings. Inhale the aromas in the air. What do you see? What do you notice? What do you feel?

As you review the menu, notice the feel of the paper, the typography, the aesthetic. Which menu items catch your eye?

As you interact with your server, be present. Engage. Make eye contact. If there's something you're curious about, ask questions. Enjoy this moment. Enjoy the experience of being served—what a luxury!

When your meal arrives, instead of immediately taking your first bite, pause. Savor the meal with your eyes, first. Take in the visual pleasure. Then savor the meal with your sense of smell. Take in the aroma. After that, slowly and appreciatively, begin to eat your meal.

Notice how flavors change and deepen as you chew. Notice how there's an intense feeling of pleasure at the beginning of your meal—that amazing first bite!—and how the pleasure-level tends to decline as your meal goes on.

When you feel satisfied—not super hungry, not super stuffed, but right in the middle—put down your fork and pause for a few minutes. Sip some water or take notes in your journal. Check in with your body after a few minutes. How do you feel?

Could you do some yoga or take a brisk walk right now?

Are you overly full, like you're about to slip into a food coma?

The goal, with this meal, is to stop eating when you feel satisfied but not overly full.

If you miss the mark at this meal—and overdo it—don't beat yourself up. It's no problem. You're going to practice eating attentively several times this week and every time you eat is another opportunity to get in tune with your body's hunger/fullness signals.

In time, it will get easier to figure out the ideal stopping point for each meal. Keep practicing.

If you'd like to record some thoughts and observations from your meal, write them down here:

_____

_____

_____

_____

_____

_____

_____

_____

Commit to eating attentively for the rest of this week—at least one meal per day. Then maybe two meals per day. Then three. Then eventually, all of your meals and snacks. The more you practice, the easier this will feel.

Food can—and should—bring you intense pleasure. Slow down so that you can soak in as much pleasure as possible. Give that gift to yourself. Your taste buds will thank you. Your digestive system and metabolism will thank you, too.

Keep practicing. Keep it slow.

Beautiful things unfold when you slow the fuck down, which I am pretty sure is a direct quote from the Buddha, y'all.

The BARE Truth

If you want a quick, five-second, snack-sized summary of this chapter, here it is:

Slow down. Eat attentively. Eat until you feel satisfied but not stuffed.

Enjoy power food. Enjoy pleasure food. Have both—in whatever proportion feels good for your body.

Continually check in with yourself to ask, "What is my body asking for today?" and "What feels like love today?"

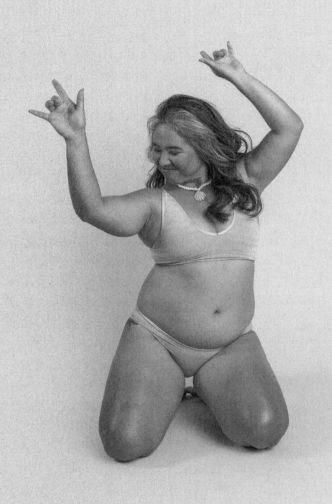

Exercise with Love

Exercise is a celebration of what your body can do—
not a punishment for what you ate.

Exercise Is Not Optional

I used to resist exercising SO MUCH. I hated it. I resented it. I thought it was boring and dumb and ditzy and even "anti-feminist." (More about all of this nonsense in a moment!)

But one day, a friend who I really respect said to me, "Susan, you have a human body, and your body was designed to move. You need to move at least three times a week. This is not optional. This is the bare minimum you need to do. This isn't about vanity. It's about your health."

As much as I grumbled, I knew she was right. A sedentary lifestyle comes with consequences. Big ones. Like a higher risk of developing cancer, heart disease, diabetes, depression . . . the list goes on and on. Not to mention, those little everyday consequences like feeling out of breath after chasing your hyperactive kid around the house for five minutes, huffing and puffing, unable to catch up. (That was totally me.)

But I don't need to tell you this. You already know that exercise is important. I probably don't need to convince you of that! The question you're probably wondering isn't *Why should I exercise?* but rather, *How can I truly commit to exercise and make it more fun?*

That's what this chapter is all about. And like so many aspects of the BARE process, it all comes back to *pleasure* and *love.*

The Big Question: What Feels Like Love?

Instead of choosing a fitness class or an exercise regime because it's "trendy" or because your favorite celebrity raves about it, tune into your body.

Ask, *What kind of movement would feel like love today?*

Your body might say to you, *I feel sluggish. I would love an energy boost. A brisk walk would be great.*

Your body might say to you, *I feel anxious and jittery. I would love an intense run or some kickboxing to uncork some of this pent-up energy.*

Your body might say to you, *Ouch, I'm super sore from yesterday's workout. Let's chill out today. Some gentle yoga sounds good.*

Unlike your brain—which can be very tricky and manipulative, inventing all kinds of wild stories about what you "need" or "deserve"—your body is much more honest. Your body never lies.

When it comes to food, and fitness, and social commitments—and everything else that goes into your body, or onto your calendar—choose whatever feels most like love. Choice by choice, the love adds up, until there's no denying the effect on your body.

Love is the ultimate personal trainer.

My Story: From Couch Potato to Marathon Runner

If you were alive in the late 1980s and early '90s, you might recall the Step Up Aerobics fitness craze. No? Allow me to refresh your memory:

Picture a dozen women wearing spandex leotards, pantyhose, leg warmers, and side ponytails stepping onto a plastic platform. Up. Down. Up. Down. Side. Side. Up. Down. Over and over. Glassy eyes and manic smiles. Stepping away to an unbelievably irritating disco beat while flapping their arms around in various configurations.

Throughout the class, the aerobics instructor would call out things like:

"Give it to me right here!"

"To the right! To the left!"

"Are we having fun yet?!"

I was a freshman student in college—majoring in journalism—during the height of the aerobics frenzy. I remember walking into a local gym, watching a class in progress, seeing the bouncing ponytails and leg warmers and thinking to myself, *Uh . . . no thanks.*

The whole thing seemed so ditsy and frivolous, and there was so much spandex.

I told myself, *Women who exercise are vain. Total bimbos. I'm too smart for this crap. I've got better things to do.*

I huffed out of the gym and vowed never to go back. Years rolled by. I did some power walking here and there to clear my mind in between classes, but aside from that, I avoided anything that even remotely resembled exercise. I was proud of this, repeatedly telling myself, *I'm not one of those bimbos who loves to work out. I'm better than that.*

Fast forward several years later, with thirty-five extra pounds on my frame, I started to wonder, *Hmmm. OK. Maybe I ought to be exercising.*

But I couldn't imagine a universe in which I—Susan Hyatt, lifelong couch potato—could become even remotely athletic.

Taking my first (very begrudging) step into exercise

At my heaviest weight, a girlfriend encouraged me to start exercising a couple times a week.

"It can be five minutes of exercise, or fifty minutes, whatever," she told me. "Just do something. Find some form of exercise that you don't completely hate, and just do it."

I begrudgingly agreed to try. At this point, I was so unhappy with my body, and so desperate, I was willing to try anything, even (gasp!) moving my body.

I chose a beginner-level Pilates DVD (remember DVDs, people?) and I started doing it three times a week in my living room. Did I enjoy it? Not particularly, at first. But it wasn't as awful as I thought it would be. Most of it involved gentle stretching and small, slow arm and leg movements. There was no leaping, jerking, or bouncing—and definitely no spandex. Thank God. There was even a whole section of the DVD where you get to lie flat on your back! "Not bad," I thought. "This, I can do."

After just a few weeks, I noticed that the Pilates movements were feeling a bit easier. Huh. I was getting stronger. Pretty exciting.

Emboldened by that discovery, I decided to add some walking into my routine. I started walking for twenty minutes a couple mornings each week. It felt good. The fresh air cleared my mind. Smart, creative ideas popped into my head, seemingly out of nowhere, almost every time I took a stroll. It was nice to wave hello to my neighbors as I circled the block. I could listen to my favorite music on my headphones, whatever I wanted to hear. This was my time. Walking became something I actually sort of looked forward to doing, not something I dreaded. Walking a couple mornings each week soon became every morning of the week. Twenty minutes of walking turned into thirty, then forty, then sixty minutes a day.

The effect was undeniable. With a combination of Pilates three times a week—plus walking every morning—I was feeling less stressed out. I slept more deeply. I had tons more energy. My digestion seemed to improve. The weight was melting off even faster. So many beautiful results—and honestly, I was barely even breaking a sweat! This wasn't some type of grueling army boot camp fitness regime. I was literally just stretching and strolling. My routine was pretty mellow as far as exercise goes. Yet it was making a noticeable difference. Who would have thunk it?

Discovering what my body can do

A couple of months after I started walking regularly, something unbelievable happened.

One day, halfway through my walk, my body started talking to me. As in, literally talking. It felt like receiving a text message from a friend.

"Why don't you start to run?" said my body.

"Huh? What now? Who dis? I don't run. I am not a runner," I snapped back.

"Well, why don't you just see?" my body nudged again.

I considered it. I assessed the situation. Currently, I was

walking briskly. Very briskly, actually. If I picked up the pace, just a teensy tiny bit, I would be jogging. I was *almost* there. Pretty close to running. Why not try?

So, I did. I started to run.

My very first thought was, *OMG! I AM RUNNING!!*

It felt preposterous. Unbelievable. I half expected the Pope to come wheeling down the street surrounded by throngs of onlookers—all gathering to witness the Divine Miracle that was unfolding, right here, on an ordinary morning in my hometown of Evansville, Indiana.

OK, BUT SERIOUSLY! I AM RUNNING!! My mind wouldn't let up. I was amazed at myself.

I decided to run as far the park. Then I could walk back home from there.

Just get to the park, just get to the park, get to the park, I kept repeating to myself.

I got to the park. And then, just as I had promised myself, I walked back home.

Back at my computer, I used Google Maps to find out approximately how far I'd been running. I was so curious. I figured I'd run a couple hundred feet. Something like that.

Nope. I had run . . . one and a half miles. I almost fainted from shock.

One and a half miles? That's, like, serious running? That's legit Olympics-level running!

The pride that I felt was like nothing I'd ever felt before. *Wow. I didn't know my body could do that.*

What can *your* body do? It's exhilarating to find out.

It Does Not Have to Be Boring

Often, my clients fear exercising ("I don't want to be the heaviest one in the class!"), feel intimidated by exercising ("I don't know what to do with all those machines at the gym!"), or have a warped attitude about exercising ("Working out is for shallow, ditzy bimbos. I have better things to do with my time"). And at first, almost all of my clients believe that exercising is going to be "sooo boring."

But it doesn't have to be! Case in point:

While leading a BARE retreat for eight clients in New York City, I told the ladies that I had a special surprise up my sleeve.

"Ooh, what?" they all wanted to know.

Ohhhhh lord. They had no idea what was coming.

"Do any of you ladies like . . . Beyoncé?" I asked, already knowing the answer. This was basically an eight-woman army of Beyoncé super-fans.

Lots of nodding and curious raised eyebrows followed.

"Well, we've been invited to take a private dance class at . . ."—pause for dramatic effect—"Beyoncé's rehearsal studio."

The squeals of glee were deafening.

We changed into tank tops and stretchy pants and cavorted over to the studio. A gorgeous choreographer named Robert Hartwell greeted us there with a huge smile. It was a stunning space—floor-to-ceiling windows with a view of the city, tons of natural light, exposed brick walls, and a ballet barre stretching from one side to the other.

"Is this the floor that Beyoncé dances on, like, for real?" I asked, feeling like a twelve-year-old girl. Robert nodded. I almost kissed the floor.

After taking approximately a million selfies and posting multiple videos on Facebook, the class began. Robert designed a routine that was perfect for beginners—not too complicated, not too fast, but totally fun and sexy—and within thirty minutes or so, we were all strutting, posing, and shimmying to the beat like professional backup dancers. (Beyoncé, if you're hiring, call us!)

All of my clients were beaming and grinning the entire time. We all broke a sweat—but nobody really felt like they were "exercising." We weren't "working out"—we were LIV-ING A DREAM!

After toweling off and hugging Robert, we went back to the hotel to gush and discuss the class. Everyone agreed that it was one of the best experiences of the whole retreat, maybe even the whole year.

"I honestly didn't realize that exercise could be that much fun!" one client exclaimed.

Yes, ma'am. It sure can.

Maybe you won't have the chance to dance in Beyoncé's studio every single day of your life (if only!), but you can find—or create—your own personal version of "dancing in Beyoncé's studio" in your own hometown. You can create that same level of "OMG THIS IS FUN!" excitement even if you live far, far away from the bright lights of NYC.

Maybe typical gym workouts bore you, and that's fine. If that's the case, skip the gym. Choose something else that feels more fun.

You don't have to settle for "boring fitness" when there are so many options out there. Choose something that makes you feel like you're heading to Beyoncé HQ. You'll enjoy the experience a lot more, and you'll be highly motivated to do it again and again.

Not sure where to begin? I've got you covered.

Tons of Exercise Options, Ideas, and Classes to Try

What's one type of exercise that sounds enjoyable? What seems interesting to you? What seems like it might feel energizing and loving for your body?

Choose something from the following list that you'd be willing to try. It doesn't matter what you choose. Just choose something and try it out—at least once. Don't like it? Try something else. Keep going until you find a style of movement that feels right for you. Please don't postpone this until later. Honor your body right now. It's yearning to move!

Aerial yoga

Do yoga poses while your body is supported by a huge, super-strong piece of fabric that's bolted to the ceiling. It feels like floating!

Aerobics

Hey, it's not my jam, but some people love it! For many it has fun, retro appeal, especially if leg warmers are involved!

Aikido

Consider this mellow form of martial arts with soft, graceful movements. In Japanese, *aikido* means "the way of harmonious spirit."

Aquarobics

If you struggle with stiff, achy joints, or if you're recovering from an injury, working out in a pool can feel really good.

Ballroom dancing

You can pretend you're a contestant on *Dancing with the Stars!*

Barre

Put your hair into a ballerina bun! Barre classes usually include lots of small movements—using the ballet barre for balance and support—so you don't have to worry about toppling over.

Belly dancing

Sensual and a seriously great workout, most belly dancing classes are very body-positive and welcoming. Bring your womanly curves here.

Boxing

Channel your inner Claressa Shields or Laila Ali. *POW!* Great way to uncork pent-up stress and feel badass as hell.

Burlesque dancing

No, you don't necessarily have to strip down and get naked . . . unless you want to! I know so many women who felt skeptical about burlesque, but after trying it, they declared it's one of the most fun, empowering things they've ever done.

Buti yoga

It's a combination of yoga postures combined with tribal-inspired dance moves, plus hip-hop vibes. If you love the idea of twerking while you're in a Downward Dog pose, this is for you.

Cardi-yoga
Try yoga mixed with heart-pumping cardio. Great choice if you've done yoga for a while and you're craving a new challenge.

Caveman workout
Build a fire using friction generated by your bare hands. Drag rocks around. Get muddy. Yes—this is a real thing. Google it. You'll find classes all over the country.

CrossFit
If you're a fairly experienced weight lifter, and you know your way around a gym, CrossFit can be a fun challenge. Beware, though: People in the CrossFit community can be intensely competitive. Folks often push way too hard—and injuries are common. So, listen carefully to your body and go at your own pace.

Curvy yoga
This is yoga designed for curvier bodies. If you feel like you "don't belong" in a typical yoga class environment, or if you feel like most yoga instructors ignore you, or don't know how to properly instruct you, you might love this. Google it. You can watch free beginner-level videos online.

Cycling

Ride your bicycle around town, just like when you were a little kid!

Hatha yoga

Release tension, stretch and elongate your muscles, and breeeeathe.

Hiking

Lace up your shoes and get out into the woods—or take an urban hike through an area of your city that you haven't explored much.

Hip-hop dancing

Channel your inner Beyoncé and shake it, mama! I took a class at Queen Bey's dance studio in NYC and it changed my life. Unforgettable. I can die happy now.

Hot yoga

Yoga with the heat cranked up! Some people love it. Some people hate it. Some people get dizzy and pass out. Proceed with caution—and bring plenty of water to rehydrate.

Kayaking

Build upper body strength while cruising down the river. Not a bad life.

Line dancing

Swing yer partner round and round! Line dancing is so hysterically funny, you'll barely even notice that you're getting a great workout.

Obstacle course

If ordinary gyms bore you to tears, maybe you'd enjoy an obstacle course? You'll find training classes and events all around the country. You'll climb ropes, scramble over boulders, and maybe even jump over burning coals. Xena the Warrior Princess would be so proud of you!

Pilates

Stretch and tone your muscles. Breathe. Chill out. For most Pilates classes, you're lying on your back the entire time— but you'll get a surprisingly good workout, nonetheless!

Pole dancing

If you think pole dancing is skanky, think again. Google "pole dance championship," watch a few YouTube videos, and prepare to have your mind blown. It's an incredible art form with gravity-defying moves. And no, you don't have to get naked.

Rock climbing

Scramble up a vertical wall and feel a rush of pride when you reach the top! You'll be safely secured in a harness in case you slip. Most rock climbing gyms also have a "kiddie wall" that's not very high or challenging, which is perfect for beginners.

Rowing

Indoor rowing is poised to be the next big fitness trend! It's a full-body workout—and you're sitting down the entire time, which means there's no intense impact on your knees or other sensitive joints.

Running

It gives you a chance to be out in nature or explore your neighborhood. Or you can hit the treadmill. Once you catch that runner's high, it's hard to stop.

Sex

Yup. It counts.

Skating

Remember the movie *Xanadu*? Channel your inner Olivia Newton John and hit the roller skating rink! Or try roller blading or ice skating.

Spinning

Spinning is another way of saying "indoor cycling." Most Spinning instructors will play loud, upbeat pop and dance music to pump up your energy.

Sports team

Baseball, basketball, soccer, ultimate Frisbee . . . there are lots of teams (for all levels) in pretty much every city. Or play with your kids. Or start your own team!

Surfing

Fresh air, sunshine, salty ocean spray . . . not a bad place to get in some exercise! Find a beginner-level surf class in your city. Or google "Surf Goddess" to find incredible surfing retreats especially for women.

Swimming

It doesn't have to be swimming laps, which plenty of people find dull. It could be water aerobics, aqua jogging, swimming in the ocean and playing in the waves, or just the thrill of splashing around.

Tai Chi

Serene, flowing movements to soothe your mind and body. Not very strenuous, but definitely very relaxing. It's like yoga on Xanax.

Tennis

Channel your inner Venus or Serena Williams and hit the courts!

Vinyasa yoga

This is one of the most common types of yoga that you'll see out there. You'll experience traditional poses—Child's pose, Warrior poses, Downward Dog—with an emphasis on correct form and deep breathing.

Walking

Left foot. Right foot. Repeat. You got this.

Weight lifting

So empowering. Great for toning your muscles and for building bone density, too. It's exciting to feel your body adapt and grow stronger. This month, maybe a ten-pound weight for that bicep curl. Next month, maybe more!

Yin yoga

Try this mellow form of yoga with super-slow-motion stretches. You'll be supported with blankets, blocks, and bolsters to get really deep into those stretches. (I've heard people jokingly call this "sleepy time yoga" or "nap yoga" because it's sooo relaxing.)

Zumba

If you like the idea of taking a dance class—but you want something beginner-friendly and accessible, with steps that are easy to follow—this might be your new jam. There are 200,000 Zumba locations worldwide—plus tons of free online videos—so you've got no excuse NOT to try this out.

Don't Want to Work Out Alone? Find Your Fitness Angel

After my very first foray into running, I felt inspired to keep going. But I knew that I needed some support and accountability to make it happen.

I asked my best friend, Frances, if she'd be willing to go for a run with me every morning. She said yes.

We've been running together—almost every single day—for the past eight years.

Running was just the beginning, too. We've had all kinds of fitness adventures together. We've tried CrossFit. We've done yoga. We've tried hiking and rowing and cycling. We didn't love every single type of exercise that we tried—some felt great, others felt awkward—but we laughed at lot, we got sweaty, we created memories, and each experience brought us even closer together. Our friendship is deeper than ever.

Frances is my Fitness Angel. She's the woman who texts me at 5 AM to say, "You up? I'm coming over for our run."

She's the woman who calls me up to say, "Uh, nope, you're coming to the gym with me tomorrow" when I feel mopey and I'm considering canceling our plans.

She's the woman who says, "Hey, have you ever tried indoor cycling? I was thinking we could give it a whirl."

Once I peed myself during a super-strenuous CrossFit class. She was the one helping me to laugh it off. "Who cares?" she told me. "Everyone pees during CrossFit. Be proud. It's a badge of honor!"

She holds me accountable to my goals. She reminds me that I'm strong when I forget that fact. She gets my butt out of bed on days when I don't think I can do it. And when she's feeling discouraged, distracted, or defeated, I do the same for her. We help each other to show up stronger in every area of our lives.

If you're thinking, "That's nice for you, Susan, but sadly I don't have a best friend like Frances. So, what am I supposed to do?"

Well, you've got options:

- You could ask one of your current friends if she'd be willing to become your workout buddy. You don't necessarily have to go running every morning at 5 AM. But maybe you could meet once a week for a mellow yoga class. Start there.

- If you have a close friend who doesn't live nearby, you could become virtual Fitness Angels for each other. Send emails with workout ideas to one another. Talk on the phone while you power walk around the neighborhood. Record an encouraging voicemail on her phone—something she can listen to when she's feeling grumpy and tired. Ask her to do the same for you. You can provide tons of support for one another even if you live multiple time zones apart.

- You could create a new friendship. In every city, of every size, I can guarantee: There are dozens (if not thousands) of women who would love to exercise more—and who would love a buddy to do it with. Go online, visit meetup .com, and find a fitness group or a running club. Or put up a flyer at your local gym that says, "Seeking: Fitness Buddy." Or post a note on Facebook. There are a million and one ways to find a Fitness Angel. One Facebook note might be all you need to do!

Claire's Story
Choosing a Gentler Option— and Losing Twenty-five Pounds

For many, deciding that exercise can be fun and pleasurable is a tough notion to wrap your head around. We're so accustomed to the idea that fitness should be punishing and grueling if we want to see real results. (That old "No pain, no gain" motto.)

"Claire" used to be the poster woman for physical punishment. She'd start her day with a brisk run to the gym, followed by a CrossFit class. In the evening, she would take another high-intensity fitness class or do another run after work. She worked out three hours a day, minimum, and was plagued with constant injuries, aches, and pains. She was such a frequent visitor at her chiropractor's office, she practically had a punch card, which she considered a point of pride.

Despite her grueling workout schedule, she was about twenty-five pounds overweight and couldn't figure out what the hell was going on. She hired me and expressed her exasperation. She wanted to know, "Why don't I look like the cover girl for a fitness magazine? I'm certainly working out like one!"

It was a mystery. After a couple of conversations, I began to suspect that her obsessive workout schedule was a cover-up for something else. Maybe she was working out like a new U.S. army recruit as a way to postpone dealing with something in her life that she didn't want to face, or because of some type of deep-rooted fear. I prodded her a bit, and she confirmed my intuition.

"Totally," she said. "I'm worried that if I stop exercising like this, I'll lose control, and I'll gain even more weight."

When clients say that they're afraid of losing control, it's usually because they already feel out of control in at least one area of life.

Maybe you feel out of control in the presence of your favorite foods, you overeat almost every night, and then you overexercise to try to erase the effects of all that excess food. Or maybe you feel powerless and out of control in some other area of your life—with your kids, your spouse, or your job, for example.

"Well, this super-intense exercise regime that you're doing isn't helping you to lose weight, is it?" I asked rhetorically.

"No."

"So, what if you try something different? Not permanently. Just for a week," I offered.

I encouraged Claire to hit pause on the grueling CrossFit schedule and try a gentler form of exercise for the next seven days.

"Maybe some yoga," I offered. "And not some kind of crazy sweat-lodge power yoga. Gentle yoga."

She agreed to try. She went to a class. Then another. And another. She hated it. The whole time, she felt like yoga was "too easy" and "a waste of her time."

But somewhere during the fourth yoga class, something happened.

The negative chattering in her mind quieted down. All of those voices saying *This is dumb* and *This doesn't count as exercise* began to fade away. Somewhere in the middle of a flowing Vinyasa sequence, she felt her body unclench and relax. She heard a voice inside of her mind—a new voice, softer and gentler than she was accustomed to hearing—say: *That's more like it.*

She was shocked. She shared the experience with me.

"It sounds like your body really enjoyed that yoga class," I told her. "How did you feel afterward?"

"Really great," she said.

"Any aches and pains, like when you do CrossFit?"

"No."

"Well, all right then. It seems pretty clear that, at least right now, your body is craving a gentler form of exercise. How about you continue doing yoga a bit longer?"

Claire felt curious to see what might happen, so she agreed to give it a whirl. Over the next several weeks, she skipped CrossFit and continued practicing yoga instead. With each gentle yoga class, her body gave her the same feedback: *Ahhhhh. Yes. That's more like it.*

Claire began to wonder, *What other areas of my life need a little more gentleness, too?*

Throughout our time together, she adjusted her morning routine. *Ahh. That's more like it.* She noticed that certain relationships in her life felt really draining, and she made some adjustments to her social circle. *Ahh. That's more like it.* Maybe mealtime could be slower and more nourishing. *Ahh. That's more like it.*

Week by week, choice by choice, Claire continued to ask herself: *What feels just right?* and *Where could I invite a little more gentleness into my life?*

Her body responded to all of these positive, loving changes, and in the process, she lost twenty-five pounds.

She couldn't believe it. All those years of punishing her body with workouts that left her bruised, swollen, or lying in pain on a doctor's table, and in the end, the big secret to losing weight was . . . a little gentleness.

The moral of this story isn't "Everybody, go take a yoga class." The moral of this story is "Listen to your body, not your fear."

That fearful, anxious inner voice might be telling you, *Run ten miles today or your weight's going to balloon up and you'll lose all control.* That voice might be a complete idiot. Challenge that voice. Listen to your body, instead.

If your body is brimming with excess energy and begging for a long run, go run.

If your body is asking for the power and confidence that weight lifting can bring, lift weights.

If your body wants to be stretched and lengthened, do a few spinal twists in a yoga class.

Try out different forms of fitness and pay attention to your body. Let your body talk to you, and really listen. Try to find that feeling of *Ahhhh. That's more like it.* When you feel that signal from within, you know you've found a type of exercise that's going to support your body instead of harming you.

Love. Care. Attentiveness. Not fear.

That's more like it.

Strong Just Like You

About five years ago, I was doing my usual morning run around the neighborhood—my BFF and running partner Frances was out of town, so on this particular morning it was just me, running solo. As I circled the corner, I noticed a cute little girl playing in her front yard. She waved at me and continued scribbling on the ground with her sidewalk chalk.

On my run back, she was standing in the same spot, but she had changed her outfit into Wonder Woman Underoos. She was jumping up and down and cheering for me. She said, "When I grow up I am gonna be strong just like YOU!" It totally made my day. I never forgot her.

Five years later, on that same morning run, I saw that same little girl—but more grown up. Several feet taller. Middle-school age. She and her mom were getting into the car.

The girl said to me, "Hey! I'm old enough to join the track team next year and I'm doing it!"

I said, "That's so awesome!"

Her mom said, "We see you almost every day, no matter the weather, out here running. You should know that my daughter always yells out, 'She's out there again!' You have inspired her through the kitchen window, most mornings."

I was rendered almost speechless. I thanked them and told them how much that meant to me.

Me—the former couch potato.

Me—the woman who used to believe that caring about physical fitness meant you were vain, shallow, or ditzy.

Me—inspiring a young woman to join the track team at school.

I went home and cried. I was bawling. Hot, happy tears streaming down my face.

What an amazing reminder that—even if you can't fathom it right now—you *can* create new habits. You *can* start exercising. You *can* find a form of exercise that feels good for you. You *can* become the type of woman who takes excellent care of herself. The type of woman who doesn't exercise because she wants to punish her body—but because she wants to celebrate what her body can do.

As you do this, you won't just be upgrading your own life—you'll become a source of inspiration for women and girls all around you.

Five years from now, you might walk, run, row, cycle, crunch, punch, lift, sprint, or dance past a young woman who looks at you and says, "When I grow up, I want to be strong just like you."

Your Assignment
Take Your Inner Athlete on a Date

This week, your assignment is to exercise three times. That's it. Pretty simple. I call this "taking your inner athlete on a date."

You can do the same workout three times. Or you can mix it up and try some different options. You can do a five-minute workout, or fifty minutes, or more. Any style, any duration, any intensity level. Whatever you want.

Once you've selected a form of exercise that you're willing to try out, get your calendar, and schedule three workouts for this week.

Three dates. Three times. Lock it into your calendar. No flaking out. This is a mandatory appointment. You will show up for yourself—and give your body some love—because you are becoming the type of woman who takes excellent care of herself.

As you're scheduling workouts into your calendar, use terminology that makes you happy. Maybe instead of "Workout," you'll put, "Body-Love Time" or "Gettin' STRONG" or "Sexy SweatFest" or "Walking Date with Karen." Use language that feels empowering to you.

After taking your inner athlete on a date three times this week, notice how you feel: Are you sleeping more deeply? Do you feel proud? Energized? Less anxious? Do you want to keep going with the type of exercise that you've chosen—or switch it up and try something else? Do you want to invite a friend to join you?

Write down some observations here.

_____

_____

_____

_____

_____

_____

_____

At the end of this week, bust out your calendar again. Schedule your three workouts for *next* week. Do this every week. This is your new normal.

Remember: Not every workout needs to be long, and not every workout needs to be strenuous. You don't necessarily need to be drenched with sweat every time. You can keep it brief and relaxed if you want to.

Any movement is better than zero movement. So just move. And keep moving.

You have one body—and you have this one lifetime to inhabit it, use it, and enjoy it.

Go discover what your body can do.

The BARE Truth

If you want a quick summary of this chapter, here it is:

Your body was born to move. This is not optional. This is mandatory. Find something that sounds pleasurable and schedule it into your life. You're not exercising to punish yourself. You're exercising because it feels good (Yes! It can feel good!) and because it's a celebration of what your body can do.

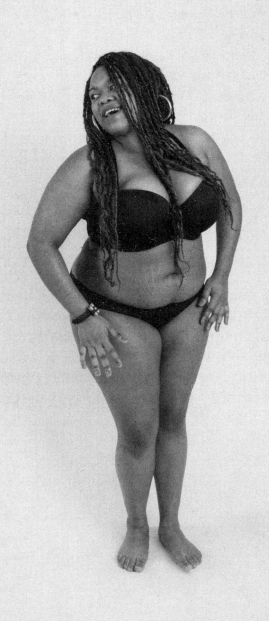

Declutter Your Closet

Your clothes influence your mood. Keep feel-good clothes in your closet—things that fit well and feel good at your current size, whatever that may be. Dress yourself like a queen.

The Story Written All Over Your Closet

If you opened my closet about twelve years ago, you might cringe. You'd see a very depressing story. You'd see pants in six different sizes—pants I was holding on to "just in case" I gained or lost weight. You'd see outdated blazers with unappealing shoulder pads. You'd see frumpy, shapeless "mom clothes" for weekends. You'd see a whole lot of "slimming" black and almost no color.

You would probably think, *This closet belongs to a woman who doesn't love the way she looks, a woman who wants to cover up and hide from the world.* And you'd be very right.

If you opened my closet today, you'd see a very different story. You'd see color. You'd see texture. You'd see shimmery sequins. You'd see dresses made for dancing. You'd see workout clothes in plain sight, not shoved away in the farthest drawer. You'd see t-shirts from trips to New York City, Paris, and Positano. Shoes that command attention. You would probably think, *This woman is living life . . . full out!*

What about you? If I were to open your closet right now, what would I see? What's the story being told? What's the message being echoed back to you every time you wake up and get dressed? Does your closet say, "Hooray! A brand-new day!" or "Ugh, not this again"?

It's time to upgrade your closet and create an inspiring, empowering environment. It's time to declutter and create some new looks for yourself—yes, even if you're not living at your ideal weight just yet.

Upgrading your closet right now will help your weight loss (or whatever type of transformation you want) move along faster. I promise.

Clothes Directly Impact How You Feel

If you hate the clothes that you're putting on when you get dressed, it affects your mood. You feel cranky. You don't feel confident. You don't feel strong and bold. Instead, you feel like hiding or disappearing. If the clothes fit poorly—if the waistband pinches you, for example—it hurts and then you get even crankier. You look in the mirror and what's reflected back at you is this message: *You're a disappointment. You don't deserve anything better than this.*

Unappealing clothes set you up for an unsuccessful day.

Now imagine the opposite scenario: If you love the clothes that you're putting on when you get dressed, it affects your mood. You feel happy. You feel confident. You feel strong and bold. You feel better about speaking up for yourself. You feel inspired to take better care of yourself. You feel comfortable, at ease in your skin. You might not be at your natural/goal weight—yet—but you're getting there! You look in the mirror and what's reflected back at you is this message: *You're beautiful. You deserve respect. You know how to take excellent care of yourself.* Maybe even, *Bow down, the Queen has arrived!*

Just like that, you've set yourself up for a highly successful day.

Coming Out of Hiding

Eight years ago, after losing a significant amount of weight—by eating attentively and by moving my body with love, not by dieting—I decided that it was time to poke around in my closet and do some decluttering. (I wish I'd done this much, much sooner.)

Most of my old clothes didn't fit anymore. Everything was several sizes too big (a nice problem to have). I opened up my closet doors, assessing the situation. I looked inside. I mean, really looked. It was like I was seeing my clothing collection with fresh eyes, for the very first time. And what I saw wasn't pretty.

If my clothing collection was a book, the title of that book would be *101 Ways to Hide Yourself.* That's what it felt like. Every single piece of clothing that I owned had been carefully selected to "hide" something about me—a part of my body, or a part of my personality.

I pulled pieces out, one by one, reflecting on why I had purchased each one:

Oh, I remember these pants. I bought these because I thought they made my ass look smaller.

Oh, wow. I forgot about this dress. I got it because the long sleeves covered my arms.

Good lord. This blazer! I bought that because I thought it made me look older and more "professional." I never even liked it, but I wanted people to respect me at work.

These weren't clothes. These were shields. These were masks. These were 101 different ways to cover up my body and my spirit.

It was a sea of beige, tan, and taupe. So many Talbots blazers, I could have opened my own store! So many Lands' End sweaters, which is what I thought a "good mom" is supposed to wear. So many garments that I never liked, that never made me feel good, that never even fit me nicely.

I dumped everything into the center of my bedroom, stood back, and stared at the massive pile of oatmeal- and camel-colored fabric. And then . . . *Ding.* An epiphany hit.

Staring at the big pile, I realized, those clothes don't belong to me. Those clothes belong to a former version of me.

This former version of me privately believed, *I am disgusting and I don't deserve to have nice things. I don't deserve to have clothes that feel good on my skin, or that I actually love.*

Those old clothes reflected that old mind-set, that old message. Those clothes were toxic.

And I needed to get them outta my house. ASAP.

I secured everything in a bag and donated the clothes to a thrift store. I knew that my discarded clothes weren't necessarily going to feel toxic for someone else. There are plenty of woman out there who genuinely love beige-colored blazers and slacks! But that woman is not me. It never was.

Most women wait until they've lost weight before they declutter their closet and discard clothes they don't like. That's what I did. But I wish I had done things differently.

I wish that I had decluttered my closet at the beginning of my weight loss journey, rather than waiting until I was nearing the end. Why? Because by hanging onto those sad, beige garments, by seeing and wearing them every day, I was bringing toxicity into my environment.

Each time I got dressed—each time I put on something that I hated—I was echoing back the message, *You don't deserve nice things. You don't deserve nice experiences. You don't deserve to own clothes that you actually enjoy wearing.*

And when you're trying to take better care of your body, that type of message is NOT helpful.

If I had decluttered my closet at the beginning of my weight loss journey, rather than waiting until the end, I suspect I would have lost weight even faster and more effortlessly.

Then I decided to test out that theory. Turns out, I was right.

Margot's Story
Black-Tie Victory

Margot desperately wanted to lose weight. She'd been trying forever without much success. On our very first phone call, I asked her, "What's the first thing you'll do once you've lost weight?"

Margot loved this question. She practically squealed with delight.

"I will go shopping! I will buy beautiful clothes. I will finally treat myself to the type of clothes that I really want. All the colors I love. Silky, sexy fabrics. My closet will be like a scene from *Sex & the City*."

"How fun!" I said. "So, your assignment for this week is to go out shopping and invest in three outfits that you love. Outfits that fit you beautifully, right now, at your current size."

Silence. Crickets. No response.

Eventually Margot replied with, "Um, what?"

I explained the assignment again. I could tell she was extremely resistant.

"No, Susan, I don't want to get new clothes now . . . I want to wait until I'm skinnier. Why buy new clothes now if I'm about to lose a bunch of weight? Doesn't make any sense!"

Except, it actually makes a lot of sense, I reasoned with Margot. I explained that upgrading your closet right now will give you a beautiful mood boost, creating positive, optimistic feelings, upgrading your whole day. I explained that when you feel really good, then you're less likely to reach for food to cope with boredom or stress. In other words, the way you dress can influence the way you eat. Finally, she agreed to try it out.

A breakthrough came a few weeks later. On the phone, Margot told me that she had attended a black-tie event.

"I bought a gorgeous floor-length dress and I had it tailored to fit me perfectly. People kept asking, 'What happened to you? What are you doing? You look amazing!'" Margot bubbled into the phone. Her voice sounded so clear and joyful. "A few months ago, I probably wouldn't have even attended that type of event. I would have declined the invitation. Because I would have felt stupid investing in a dress like that."

Margot has lost a significant amount of weight since beginning the BARE process. That black-tie gown doesn't fit her anymore. She's down to a smaller size—and she gave the gown away to a friend. It served its purpose in her life, and she felt completely happy to pass it along to a new home.

I've seen Margot's story play out, over and over, with so many of my clients. It's always the same story line:

I encourage my client to declutter her closet and invest in a few outfits that she loves. She says, "No, that's silly." I insist that it's a good idea and explain why. She reluctantly agrees to try.

Then she quickly discovers how good it feels to purge dowdy, depressing clothes from your closet, and how good it feels to invest in a few outfits that you're actually excited to wear. She feels better right away—which makes it that much easier to eat attentively, to exercise with love, and to take excellent care of herself in every way because she's already proven she'll treat herself with the respect she deserves.

She loses weight. And then she thanks me later.

How to Decide What to Keep in Your Closet—and What to Release

Recently, after reading Marie Kondo's best-selling book, *The Life-Changing Magic of Tidying Up*, I felt inspired to declutter my closet yet again.

If you've never read Kondo's book, it's a lovely guide to creating a serene, harmonious home filled with possessions you love. In the book, she urges you to physically touch every single item that you own—every fork, every book, every sock—and ask yourself, *Does this spark joy?*

If it sparks joy, then it stays. If it doesn't spark joy, then it's got to go.

So, into my closet I went, ready to discern which clothes sparked joy and which did not. Ready to Kondo it up, big time.

It was a surprising experience. All of my clothes fit me nicely. All of the larger-sized clothing had been purged years ago. And all of my clothes were very pretty. But there were quite a few items that I never, ever wore but that I'd been holding on to—for years—because "it was on sale" or "it was such a good deal" or "it's flattering" on my body, even though I don't particularly love it. There was nothing "wrong" with these items—but they didn't spark any feelings of joy. Into the "donate" pile they went!

It felt good to let those items go, and the experience reminded me that there's always something else you can let go.

To declutter your closet effectively, it's good to come up with a specific question that you can use to determine what stays and what goes.

Here are some questions to consider:

Does this spark joy?

This is the question that Marie Kondo, a decluttering professional, encourages her clients to ask. If a piece of clothing sparks a feeling of joy, keep it. If it doesn't spark joy, trash it, recycle it, donate it, swap it, or sell it. Just get rid of it.

Does this make me feel like I am flying in first class or coach?

A friend mentioned this question to me, and I love it! To me, the phrase "first class" indicates luxury, attention to detail, a special experience that feels like a fabulous treat. Do those old, stained, stretched-out panties make you feel like you're flying in first class? Uh. Probably not. Byeee.

Does this make me feel _____?

Insert your word of choice here. Maybe your number-one goal right now is to feel sexy, confident, relaxed, powerful, vibrant, affluent, compassionate, serene, or . . . something else? Choose a word (or a couple of words) to describe how you want to feel. Then declutter your clothes accordingly. If something doesn't make you feel the way you want to feel, toss it.

Joyce's Story
Releasing the Pantsuits

"Joyce" felt morally conflicted about decluttering her closet, which was filled with corporate-looking power suits from the early 1980s. Picture a sea of shoulder pads, gigantic buttons, and outdated cuts. All of the suits were several sizes too small for her, at her current weight, and she didn't even like the styles very much. Besides, she wasn't working in corporate America anymore. She had recently started her own business, and she could wear whatever she wanted, so there was absolutely no need to hold on to those old suits. Except . . .

"Everything is designer!" she told me, with a panicked tinge to her voice.

"What if you donated all of those suits to a charity organization, like Dress for Success?" I asked. "I'm sure a woman who's going through a difficult time, financially, would be thrilled to have a designer suit to wear to her next job interview. That suit could open doors for her. It could change her life."

Joyce mulled it over. She could see my point, and she liked the idea of helping another woman to land a job. But . . . something was stopping her. Every time she walked over to her closet to start the decluttering process, she felt so resistant—like an invisible wall was holding her back. Why?

We talked about it during our next coaching session. Gradually, we unraveled the mystery. Joyce hadn't initially realized it, but to her, these designer suits represented a former time in her life—a time when she was thinner and younger, had a prestigious job title, and earned an enviable salary to match. A time when she felt like she had it all together. She yearned to return to that time. By getting rid of the suits, she would have to admit to herself, *That particular chapter of my life is over.* She didn't want to do that.

Through our conversations, Joyce began to see that clinging to the past isn't helpful or healthy. There's no time travel machine that's going to carry you back to the 1980s, no matter how many shoulder pads you keep in your closet. It was time for Joyce to release the past, embrace the present, and focus on the future.

It took some coaxing, but she finally did it. She got rid of the suits. Every last one. Her closet was practically empty. It felt thrilling, and a little bit scary, to stare into that empty space. It was a blank canvas waiting to be filled.

Following my recommendation, she went out and purchased three new outfits that she really loved and couldn't wait to wear. Three outfits that reflected the woman she is today, not the woman she was almost thirty years ago.

Decluttering her closet felt like shedding the costumes of the past. She looked and felt better, physically, and there was an interesting financial side effect, too: She fully committed to her new business and started enthusiastically talking about her work and marketing herself. It was as if she came out of hiding.

Joyce went from having almost no clients to having more clients than she knew what to do with. In one of our later coaching sessions, we spent most of the hour talking about how to successfully manage this new influx of clients—which is a very "happy problem" to have!

It's amazing how much can change when you purge toxic clothes from your closet, stop living in the past, and step bravely into the present.

Concerns You May Have

There can be a lot of resistance around decluttering your closet and treating yourself to some new clothes. Here are some objections I frequently hear:

What if I declutter my closet and then I have nothing left?

Honestly, that's OK. It's better to have three, four, five, or six outfits that you truly like than thirty outfits that you don't like and that make you feel bad about yourself.

It's fine to strip your closet down to the bare essentials. With three to six outfits, and a few pairs of shoes and accessories, you can do a lot of mixing and matching and create a lot of different looks. You might not need as many clothes as you think you do.

Bottom line: Why hold on to clothes that don't make you feel good? If it's sending you a negative, exhausting message, then it's toxic. It's got to go.

Shouldn't I hold on to my larger clothes in case I gain back some weight?

After dumping all of my beige and taupe clothes into the center of my bedroom years ago, I wrestled with this question.

Was it really prudent to get rid of everything I used to wear at my heavier size? Like, everything-everything? What if I gained weight again at some point in the future? Wouldn't it be smart to have a few pieces around just in case?

Ultimately I decided, *No. Everything has got to go.*

I knew if I kept those bigger sizes in my closet, those clothes would send a message to me every day. And it was a powerfully toxic message: *All these positive, loving changes that I've made won't last. I don't trust myself.*

I don't want that in my environment, in my closet, and certainly not on my skin in the form of a shirt or a dress.

At this point in the BARE process, you've already cleaned up your environment, tossing out media and relationships that are harming you. And you've felt the boost in that. Your closet is one of the biggest parts of your environment, and decluttering will make such a big change for your well-being.

Enjoy the fresh, open space that you've cleared for yourself. You've opened up more space for love and pleasure to pour in.

What if I can't afford to shop for new clothes right now?

If you're on a tight budget, you can head to thrift stores, you can hunt for deals online, you can swap clothes with friends, or you can sell old clothes at vintage stores in exchange for cash or store credit. There's always a way to find something appealing—on any budget.

One client of mine was working with an extremely limited budget. She really, truly could not afford to purchase three brand-new outfits. So, she improvised. She took a shapeless dress from her closet—something she already owned that she didn't particularly love—and she added a cute belt that she'd found in the discount bin at a thrift store. *Voilà!* The baggy dress now looked flattering and super chic—and she felt excited to wear it.

Also, you don't have to keep buying new clothes. I am not asking you to purchase 100 new outfits every time you lose one pound. That would be financially ridiculous. I am encouraging you to purchase three outfits—just three for starters—that you like, that feel good on your skin, and that suit your current size.

Your Assignment
Declutter Your Closet and Shop for Three Outfits

If you feel like you can't declutter your entire closet in one week, then break things into stages. Start with something that doesn't feel too intimidating—maybe a sock drawer. Then move along to another section. Keep going.

And if the idea of going through your closet—alone—feels totally overwhelming, get help. Enlist a friend to help you out. Or get your kids involved. Or hire a professional decluttering expert if that works for your budget. It might not be as costly as you think. You can go to a website such as TaskRabbit.com and find a cleaner/organizer/helper for around $20 an hour. They'll even take your trash and donation bags and clear 'em out of your house! Hooray!

Keep whittling things down until you're left with clothes that you genuinely like—items that bring you joy, pleasure, a spark of happiness.

Then take yourself shopping and get (at least) three new outfits that you like—and that fit you well at your current size. Remember, it's better to have three outfits that "work" right now rather than 100 outfits that you hate or that don't fit. With a little creativity, you can take three outfits and do some mixing, matching, and accessorizing to create a lot of different looks!

And it goes without saying, but I'll say it anyway . . . be very gentle with yourself. Be kind. Digging into your closet is a big thing—and it might bring up a lot of emotions about your body, your weight, and your past struggles with food, about money and past spending, about choices you've made.

Keep reminding yourself, *All of that stuff is in the past. It happened. I learned plenty of things about myself. And I'm moving beyond it. I am revamping my closet now to celebrate the new me—the woman I'm becoming.*

Notice how things feel as you revamp your closet. Do you feel lighter? Happier? Liberated? Are there any other emotions bubbling up? Maybe it feels tough to let go of certain items—or maybe not. Maybe you're feeling inspired to put together all kinds of new outfits by repurposing garments that you'd forgotten all about. Maybe you had an epiphany about your marriage while you were reorganizing your underwear drawer. Record your observations here.

_____

_____

_____

_____

_____

_____

_____

_____

The BARE Truth

A quick summary of this chapter, in case you want a five-second refresher:

When you declutter your closet, it's a powerful step forward into the body and life that you want.

You're not just getting rid of old clothes. You're discarding old messages, old belief systems, and corrosive myths about what kind of woman you are.

You're stripping away the physical and emotional gunk that is weighing you down. You're saying: *I trust myself to continue moving forward on this journey. I don't need these old things anymore. Because I'm not going backward. Only forward.*

Keep stripping until your closet looks like the type of closet that belongs to a woman who treats herself with excellent care, and who is moving forward into a bright, delicious future.

Then invest in a few new outfits that you love and that fit you well. These clothes will send a new kind of message to you: "You're a woman who can have beautiful things in your closet and in your life. Not someday later. Right now."

Let *that* be the message you see every time you open those doors to get dressed. Let *that* be the message that you wear on your bare skin.

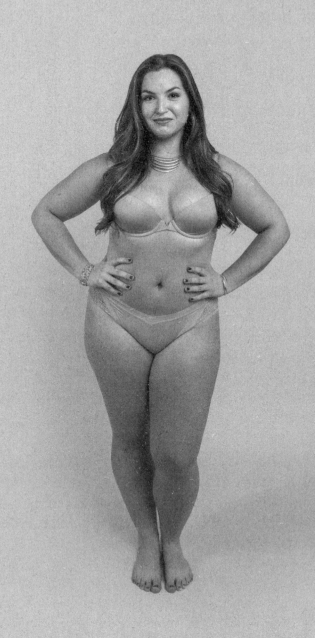

Detox Your Mind

Some thoughts energize you.
Some thoughts exhaust you.
It's time to clear out the exhausting thoughts
that are weighing you down.

What's Happening Inside Your Head?

I live near a cathedral with a bell tower that chimes every hour.

Each time I hear the bell, I pause whatever I'm doing for a moment, and I ask myself, *What am I thinking?* I try to capture my last couple of thoughts before they slip away. It's kind of like eavesdropping on my own mind.

I've been doing this little hourly ritual for more than eleven years. That said, I don't do it every single hour of my life, but when I'm working from my home office near the cathedral, I do it pretty consistently.

Eleven years ago, when I first started doing this hourly check-in, it was shocking. My thoughts were intensely negative. Almost violent. Every hour, when I heard the cathedral bell go "bong," I would eavesdrop on myself for a few moments and I would discover a barrage of self-criticism—so vicious and cruel, I almost couldn't believe it was coming from inside my own mind.

Bong. If people knew the real me, they wouldn't like me.
Bong. I am not that talented at anything.
Bong. I am a terrible parent.
Bong. I am a bad person.
Bong. I am so selfish.
Bong. My kids would be better off with a different mom.

One day, I decided to write down my thoughts once per hour. At the end of the day, I read the entire list back to myself. I remember thinking to myself, *Good lord! With thoughts like those, no wonder I feel exhausted all the time!*

And with thoughts like those, no wonder I was stuffing down my sadness with ice cream, nachos, chips, and mid-day margaritas. The negativity inside my head was deafening. It was like I had a mean, snarky teenage girl inside my mind, bullying me on an hourly basis. Anyone who gets bullied like that is bound to seek any available comfort. Who wouldn't?

Shortly after that experience, I discovered a woman named Byron Katie and her book, *Loving What Is.* In this book, Katie shares an idea that, quite literally, changed my life: *You don't have to believe all of your thoughts.*

She goes on to explain that thousands of thoughts pop into your head all day long. Some thoughts are true. Some thoughts are untrue. Some feel true for you, but they might not necessarily feel true for everyone around you. Some thoughts energize you. Some thoughts exhaust you. Some thoughts help you to work productively and take your life in the direction you want. Some thoughts hold you back.

So many different thoughts, floating through your mind like clouds passing through the sky. But you don't have to believe all of them. And you don't have to keep all of them. You can choose to keep certain thoughts, and you can choose to let other thoughts go.

Just like you can declutter your environment or your closet, you can declutter your mind—stripping away anything that weighs you down. When you find yourself in the middle of a negative, stressful, or exhausting thought, Katie urges you to ask yourself the following four questions:

Is it true?

Can you absolutely know that it's true? (Are you 100 percent certain? Could you prove it in a court of law?)

How do you react, and what happens, when you believe that thought?

Who would you be without this thought?

When you take yourself through these four questions, you usually decide, *I would be better off if I stopped believing this thought.* And then you can take steps to let it go.

Just Because a Thought Crosses Your Mind Doesn't Mean It's True

Discovering Byron Katie's work felt like getting a new pair of glasses. I could see the world in an entirely new way, and new things snapped into focus. It was a reality-altering concept for me: *I don't have to believe all of my thoughts.*

I decided to work through the four questions that Katie lays out. I was curious to see what I'd discover about myself.

One thought that I had almost constantly back then was *I am fat and disgusting.* That thought popped into my head about a dozen times a day. I decided to unravel that thought using Katie's approach.

I took this thought—*I am fat and disgusting*—and I put it through the four questions:

Is it true?

Yes. It's true. I have gained thirty-five pounds and I hate how I look.

Can you absolutely know that it's true? (Could you prove it in a court of law?)

Yes. Well, actually . . . hmm. Some people might not agree that I'm disgusting. My husband doesn't feel that way. My kids don't feel that way. There are plenty of people who might even describe me as "beautiful." And I am not the fattest person on planet Earth. If I was standing before a judge and jury, they might not agree that I am "a disgusting person." So, maybe it's not "universally true." It just feels true for me.

How do you react, and what happens, when you believe that thought?

What happens is . . . I feel awful. I feel ashamed for letting myself go. I feel scared. I feel hopeless. I feel like I want to curl up under a blanket and hide from the world.

Who would you be without this thought?

If thinking "I am fat and disgusting" was no longer a part of my day, I would feel so light and free. I would feel more peaceful. I would feel less anxious. I would be a different person.

Answering those four questions was illuminating. I realized that this recurring thought—*I am fat and disgusting*—is hurting me and exhausting me. This thought is making it *harder* for me to lose weight, not *easier.*

I just need to figure out how to get it out of my mind. But how? How do you take out the garbage when the garbage is inside your mind? It's not like a sweater you can donate, or a book you can toss into a recycling bin. It's . . . inside. So, how?

Taking Out the Garbage:
How to Deal with Toxic Thoughts

I didn't know how. So, I started studying.

It took years of therapy, life coaching, personal trial and error, and going through a master's level life coaching certification program (more than 1,000 hours of training) before I found some workable solutions.

As if turns out, there's not just one correct way to deal with toxic thoughts. You've got lots of options. You can reframe it. You can talk back to it. You can try a variety of other approaches, too.

Here are six different ways that you can deal with a toxic thought—basically, six different ways to "take out the garbage."

Reframe it

When you reframe a thought, you describe that same thought but with different wording, and from a more compassionate, encouraging perspective.

Thought:	*I am fat and disgusting.*
Translation:	*It's true that I am heavier than I'd like to be. I am not comfortable at this size. That's why I am learning how to eat more attentively, how to exercise with love, and how to strip everything out of my life that's weighing me down. I'm on a weight-loss journey. I still have a ways to go, but I am moving in the right direction, and I can already see and feel the results of my work.* (compassionate, encouraging thought)

Turn it

When you turn a thought around, you change the wording to reverse it—so that now, you're thinking the opposite of your original thought. You can also remove a word and replace it with a different word to create a new thought that feels more helpful to you. (Byron Katie teaches a version of this technique in her book *Loving What Is.*)

Thought: *I am a horrible person.*
Turnaround: *I am not a horrible person.* (opposite thought)
              My thoughts are horrible. (replacing "I" with "My thoughts")

Grab it

A woman named Nicole Antoinette came up with this technique. It's adorable and very effective!

If you sense a harmful thought running through your mind, trampling over your mood, dragging mud everywhere and mucking up your day, pretend that thought is a cute little puppy. (Puppies don't "mean" to do naughty, destructive things. But sometimes they get loose and skitter around . . . out of control!)

Grab the thought and say, "No!" Then carry the puppy to its bed, crate, or outside playpen area. Set it down. Pet its fluffy head. Remind the puppy that it's not allowed to run wild inside your mind like that. Stay. Good dog.

Thought: *I will never lose this weight. I can't succeed.*
Puppy reply: *No! That is not how we behave. You cannot run wild with this negativity. Now sit still! Stay. And be good.* (training your runaway thought)

Alchemize it

There are nuns and monks who practice a form of meditation called Tonglen meditation. It's a beautiful practice.

You breathe in deeply. You imagine that you're inhaling all of the world's suffering, including your own suffering. You can imagine that you're breathing in dark, murky air. An inky black color.

Then you exhale powerfully. You imagine that—through the power of your strong, compassionate heart—you are alchemizing all of that darkness and turning it into pure white light. You exhale white light back out into the world, encircling yourself and all living beings with love.

Inhale suffering. Exhale love. Inhale darkness. Exhale light.

I love this form of meditation. To me, it feels very empowering. With every breath, it's like saying to yourself, *I have the power to convert a negative feeling into a positive one,* and *I can turn a dark, challenging moment into an opportunity to give myself, and others, even more love.*

Thought: *I fail at everything, and I'm going to fail at this, too.*

Meditation: *Inhale your suffering and your sense of failure. Exhale love and a sense of accomplishment. Inhale darkness. Exhale love.*

Punch it

Grab a pillow. Go into a private room. Close the door. Punch that pillow while vocalizing your feelings out loud. There's some real proof behind this technique. A colleague of mine, Dr. Suzanne Gelb, is a psychologist who studied this "pillow-punching technique" as part of her PhD dissertation. She has found that it is one of *the* most effective ways to get harmful emotions out of your body, within just a few minutes. She also says that many of her clients resist trying it—because it seems silly, or they're worried someone will discover them. But when clients finally give it a try, they're usually pretty astounded at how effectively it works.

If you have wrist issues, instead of punching the pillow with your bare hand, you can thwack it with a towel. Same effect. If you like the idea of punching, but you don't want to do it at home because you don't have any privacy, consider signing up for a boxing class at your local gym. It's not exactly the same, but you'll get a similar effect.

Thought: *I am so sick of being fat! or I hate feeling this way!*

Punch it: *Thwack a pillow while you voice your frustrations out loud. After a few minutes of punching, you may notice a "shift" in your body. You might feel relaxed, light, and clear, like you've just purged your mind of something really heavy. You might even start to giggle or cry. Let it all out.*

Disprove it

If you continually think to yourself, *I am lazy* (or any kind of disempowering thought), you can gather evidence to oppose that thought and prove to yourself that it isn't true.

Thought: *I am lazy.*

Present   *Actually, that's not true. I took a beautiful walk*
evidence: *yesterday and moved my body for thirty minutes. I'm heading out for another walk right now. Just watch me.*

Thought:	*I am selfish.*
Present evidence:	*That's totally inaccurate. I wrote a beautiful thank-you note to my best friend this morning, just to let her know how much I treasure her presence in my life. She's going to be so happy when she receives that note in the mail. Would a "selfish" person do something like that? I don't think so.*
Thought:	*I can't stop binge-eating.*
Present evidence:	*Nope. Not true. I felt the urge to binge-eat a carton of pudding last night, but I chose not to act on that impulse. I chose to give my body some love, instead of stuffing/harming myself. So, I've proven to myself that I am capable of choosing love. I've done it in the past, and I can do it again.*

Shelve it

Sometimes, when a harmful thought pops into your mind, you're just not in a position to deal with it at that exact moment. Maybe you're in the middle of an important meeting at work. Or a job interview. Or you're taking care of your child or your elderly parent. Or something else that demands your full attention. In instances like those, it's OK to take the negative emotion that you're feeling and "put it on the shelf"—that is, temporarily set it aside for a few hours until you're in a position where you can effectively deal with it.

Putting a feeling "on the shelf" is not the same thing as "suppressing" a feeling. You're not pretending that everything is OK when it's really not. You're not lying to yourself or plastering on a fake happy smile. You're just choosing to process and deal with that feeling a bit later.

Later, when you return to that feeling, you typically discover that it has "simmered down" a bit. It doesn't feel quite
as overwhelming as it did a few hours earlier. You're calmer
and better equipped to choose your next move.

Let's say my son, Ryan, texts me to say, "Mom, I got sus-
pended from school. I'm at home with Dad now." I receive this
text in the middle of an important meeting with a client. I feel
sick to my stomach. I feel angry at Ryan and angry at myself.
But rather than canceling my meeting and rushing home, I
can set my feelings "on the shelf" (basically, on an imaginary
bookshelf inside my mind). I can attend to those feelings later.

Thought:	*I am a bad mom.* (when hearing about how your child has misbehaved in the middle of a busy day)
Put it on the shelf:	*I don't have time to unpack this emotion now. It is going up on my imaginary shelf. I can address these negative feelings later when I have a moment to myself.*

Bounce it

Personally, this is my favorite technique for dealing with
toxic thoughts. I love talking back to my thoughts, challenging them, and sometimes, simply demanding that they leave
me alone. (Oh, yes—I kick thoughts out of my own head all
the time, like a bouncer kicking creeps and hooligans out of
a nightclub.)

Thought:	*I am fat and disgusting.*
Bounce it:	*Oh, this thought again? You're trying to sneak past me to get inside my head and my heart. Well, no deal. This is a space for positive thoughts, and you are being ejected from the premises. You can go now.*

No One Is Completely Free of Negativity

No one's mind is 100 percent negativity-free. Everyone has negative, harmful, toxic thoughts from time to time. Even Buddhist monks who meditate on mountaintops all day long. Even professional life coaches who teach positivity for a living. Everyone is human.

Personally, I have these types of thoughts every single day of my life! Much, much less frequently than I once did. But occasionally, they still weasel their way into my mind.

As far as I know, it's not possible to completely scrub negative thoughts out of your mind. But you can work on reducing negative thoughts a lot, and you can work on managing them more effectively when they do come up.

Gloria's Story
Change Doesn't Always Have to Be "Hard"

Gloria is a driven, perfectionistic, high-achieving woman. When she sets a goal, she nails it. When she wants something, she gets it. She was raised with a puritanical work ethic and was taught, from an early age, "If it's not 'hard,' then it's not a worthy goal."

Losing weight was the one goal she hadn't been able to conquer. So, naturally, she assumed it was because she wasn't working "hard" enough. She didn't realize it when we initially met, but this recurring thought—*Change needs to be really HARD*—was hindering her weight-loss progress and making her life feel pretty miserable.

During one of our coaching sessions, I checked in to see if she was practicing mindful, attentive eating.

"Are you eating more slowly, taking time to relax and savor your meals?" I asked. "How's that going?"

"Not good," she replied. In fact, she hadn't really tried this at all, because she rejected the whole idea that "eating attentively" would help her to lose weight. Why? Because it sounded too gentle. Too easy. In her mind, change was supposed to be "hard." Not easy.

"I'm the kind of person . . ." she explained, ". . . who really needs a structured meal plan to follow. I don't do well when there's no structure. I need a plan."

I told her, "You've got a plan. The 'plan' is that you'll tune into your body and ask, 'What feels like love?' and then feed yourself accordingly."

She scoffed at this, telling me that she needed a "real plan" for her meals and also an exercise plan that was "hard as shit" (those were her exact words) or nothing was ever going to change. From the insistent tone in her voice, I could tell that this was a deeply ingrained belief that would be difficult to dissolve. I needed to take the conversation in a new direction.

"Gloria, can you think of a moment in your life when a 'big change' happened with ease?" I asked. "For example, when your child was born, was it 'hard' to love your child? Did you have to 'work' at it? Or did it happen naturally?"

This question caught her off-guard. She admitted that loving her child was easy, not "hard work." It felt natural. It just happened.

"Is it possible, then, that loving your body and taking good care of your body could feel easy and natural, too? Just like loving your child?"

She admitted, yes, maybe that's possible, too. This dialogue changed the entire tone of our conversation.

Gloria began to wonder aloud, "Maybe 'changing' doesn't always have to be so 'hard.' Maybe sometimes, big things can happen in my life and it can feel gentle, natural, even easy."

Week by week, we worked on dismantling the erroneous belief that "change needs to be hard." And week by week, Gloria began to lose weight.

"I have a habit of making things so hard for myself," she told me, several weeks into our work together. "And I always push myself so hard. But maybe I can ease up. Maybe that's the piece that's been missing all these years."

We all walk around with our minds packed with various thoughts. Some are true. Some are false. Some "seem" true, but aren't actually true, or aren't true in every scenario.

If you have a recurring thought, such as *Change needs to be HARD* or *Taking care of my body is HARD* or *Eating well is HARD,* try challenging that thought, like Gloria did. Can you find evidence to prove that, in at least some instances, the opposite of this thought might be true as well?

You get to choose what to believe, and you can choose to believe something that's going to make your life feel better, instead of making your life so much harder than it needs to be.

Cassandra's Story
What Are the Facts?

"Cassandra" was raised in a family that placed an extremely high value on weight and physical appearance. In her family, if you were thin, that meant you were successful. If you weren't thin, you were a failure, regardless of your other positive attributes. Never mind your personality, your spirit, your kind heart, or your creative talents. Your weight was the main thing that mattered.

On a phone call with me, Cassandra felt brave enough to share her greatest fear: "I'm scared that if I get fatter, everyone will stop loving me, and everyone will leave me. My husband, my kids, everyone. Nobody will want to be around me."

This fearful thought was so dominant in Cassandra's mind, it was like a terrifying specter, haunting and harassing her. She had this thought multiple times a day, maybe multiple times an hour. She lived in a continual state of anxiety and dread. She'd recently gained some weight, and this only amplified her fear and made her feel awful, which led her to overeat, which in turn caused more weight gain, which made her feel even more terrified. And so, the cycle continued.

"Is it actually true?" I asked her, during one of our coaching sessions. "This fear that you have—that everyone will stop loving you if you gain more weight—is it actually true?"

She was conflicted. Maybe. Probably.

"Well, let's look at the evidence," I said. "Your husband loves you and tells you so, daily. Your kids think the world of you. Your friends care about you. Your colleagues at work think you're wonderful. You've gained some weight recently—in fact, you're at your heaviest weight ever—and has anybody stopped loving you? Has one single person stopped?"

"No," she admitted, through tears and sniffles.

"So, what does that evidence say to you?"

"Even if I gain weight, that doesn't mean everybody will stop loving me. Nobody is leaving."

Bingo. It was a breakthrough moment for Cassandra—a moment where she realized that even if your "emotions" say one thing, the "evidence" from your life might tell a completely different story.

In the weeks that followed, she returned to that "evidence" whenever she felt anxious, and it calmed her, helping her to take care of her body in a much kinder way, which actually led to weight loss.

You might be mired in a whirlwind of fear and anxiety, fearing that something horrendous is going to happen if you "get fatter," but when you step back and look at the facts, you might realize that's simply not true.

Don't doubt that the people who really love you truly do love you. Period. And anybody who "stops" loving you because of your weight doesn't deserve to be part of your life.

You Are in Charge of Your Thoughts

If you've ever had a chance to meet one of your personal heroes, you know that it's an intensely emotional experience. You feel elated, but also nervous and jittery. You're praying you don't do something embarrassing. You're worried about how your breath smells. You're fidgeting with your bra strap, trying to will yourself to stop perspiring.

Imagine that you're about to meet your number-one hero. But that's not all: Your hero is going to meticulously review your work and give you constructive criticism, in public, in front of a classroom filled with your peers. Um . . . jitters times infinity.

That's exactly what happened for me while I was enrolled in a life-coach certification program. My personal hero—the legendary Martha Beck, a best-selling author and one of my all-time favorite writers—was teaching a writing class. The topic: How to write inspiring articles in the self-help/personal development genre. It was like taking a class on compassion from Mother Teresa herself. I felt like I was in the presence of a true master, a living legend. And I was.

For my writing assignment, I wrote an article on what to do—as a parent—when your child is diagnosed with attention deficit hyperactivity disorder (ADHD). I'd been through this exact saga with my son, Ryan, so I wrote from my own personal experiences. I also did some research to compile a list of holistic options for parents who don't necessarily want to put their child on medication. I thought my article turned out pretty nicely. I turned it in to Martha, crossing my fingers for good luck.

Then came review day. Martha reviewed everyone's articles, one by one, in front of the entire class. For each article, she gave a few pieces of praise followed by some constructive criticism, plus some ideas on how to make the article even stronger. Each student nodded, scribbling down notes, eager to improve.

Finally, it was my turn. I could barely breathe. The whole thing felt surreal. My hero, my favorite author, about to review my little article. My heart pounded in my chest. Already, I could feel the negative emotions rushing in: *You should have chosen a different topic. She's going to rip you apart. You're not as good a writer as you think you are.*

Martha began to talk about my article. And she gushed with praise. She told the class how excellent it was, how it was a perfect example of how to construct a self-help article effectively, and how there's really nothing she would change.

"Great work, Susan."

Uh. What?

I waited a few beats, assuming that the torrential down-pour of criticism was coming next. Surely there was some-thing "wrong" with my article? Nope. Martha moved on to the next lesson topic. Apparently, she had nothing more to say about my article. I was stunned.

After the writing class was over, I found myself back in my kitchen at home, pacing back and forth across the tiles, grappling with what had just happened. My brain was swirl-ing with dozens of thoughts, ranging from jubilant to anxious to intensely toxic:

OMG! I did it! I wrote a really good article and Martha loved it!

But maybe it wasn't really that good. Maybe she was just being gentle with me.

No, it was really good! But what if, next time, I write something really crappy? Now the standards are too high. What if, next time, I let her down?

What if that one article was all I got? What if my creativity is all used up now? What if I can't ever write something that good again?

At this point in my life, I had lost thirty-five pounds and my relationship with food—and my body—was vastly improved. I was in a pretty positive place. But the experience with Mar-tha and the writing class triggered a torrential downpour of negative inner chatter. I felt like it was too much to handle.

Almost unconsciously, as if I was sleepwalking, I found myself opening the fridge and peering inside, searching for cream, cheese, and butter. I was thinking to myself, *It's been a really intense day. I need fettuccini alfredo. I need mashed potatoes with butter. I need fried chicken. I want a big meal that's going to comfort me. I deserve it.*

I was reaching for the butter. I was mentally rolling through recipes in my mind. I was fully prepared to cook a gigantic feast and, quite possibly, binge-eat my way through the entire thing. If this was a horror movie, this would be the scene where you're yelling at the screen, saying, "No, lady! Don't go down into the basement! He's inside the house!! Back away!!"

Then I woke up.

It literally felt like snapping awake from a dream. I dropped the butter. I shut the fridge door. I thought to myself, *What the hell? What just happened to me?* And I backed away and got the hell out of the kitchen.

I took a few deep breaths. That was a close call. I realized just because I've made a huge amount of progress with my body—and my life—that doesn't mean that I am done with this work. There are still going to be moments where my emotions feel like too much to handle. In those moments, I need to stay awake. I need to be extra attentive. I need to give myself extra love.

I returned to my favorite question: "What feels like love?" And that night, instead of gorging on creamy pasta until I felt sick, I was able to give my body the kind of love it really craved. I took a walk to uncork some pent-up energy. I took a bath. I enjoyed a nourishing meal with my family. I wrapped up my day feeling relaxed and optimistic, rather than ending my day in an uncomfortable food coma.

That experience reminded me, yet again, that when a thought pops into your mind—like, *Eat a pound of pasta because you deserve it*—you don't necessarily have to believe that thought, and you certainly don't have to act on that thought.

You can choose which thoughts to keep and which thoughts to evict from your mind. You are not powerless in the face of your emotions. You get to choose.

I am proud, in that moment, that I was able to choose "loving myself" rather than "overstuffing myself" or "harming myself" with a boatload of pasta and fried chicken.

You can make that same choice, too. Sometimes it's easy to make the loving choice. Other times it requires grit and strength. But it's always doable.

Even when you're leaning into the yellow glow of your fridge, wrapping your fingers around a stick of butter, or a canister of frosting, or a tube of cookie dough, you can stop yourself before you fall off the ledge. You can back away and say,

"Not this time. I choose love."

Your Assignment
Eavesdrop on Your Thoughts for One Day

This week, your assignment is to eavesdrop on your thoughts for one day.

I recommend setting a timer that goes off once an hour. When it goes off, check in: What's happening in your brain? What were you just thinking?

Whatever it is, write it down. This assignment is all about building awareness—becoming aware of the kinds of thoughts that run through your mind each day.

Most likely, you will discover a lot of crappy thoughts. You may even notice that certain thoughts keep coming up again and again. Repeat offenders!

Some very common repeat offenders for my clients are:

I am fat and disgusting.

I'm never going to be able to lose weight.

I screwed up.

I feel so ashamed of myself.

I hate my body.

I hate how I look.

I have no willpower.

I am out of control.

I'm not strong enough.

I'm not smart enough.

I'm not patient enough.

I can't do this.

I never finish anything.

I'm a lazy person.

I'm a selfish person.

I'm a bad mom.

I'm a bad wife.

I've wasted so much of my life.

It's too late for me to change.

I'm pathetic.

If people knew the "real me," they wouldn't like me.

I'm sick.

I'm a monster.

All I want you to do—this week—is eavesdrop on your thoughts for a day and see what you discover. Simply building awareness is a big step.

But if you'd like to take this assignment a bit further, then the next step is to choose a toxic thought and work on clearing it out. Remember, you've got lots of different options to do this. (Revisit page 156 of this book to refresh your memory. For example, you can reframe the thought. You can disprove it. You can punch it out. You can boot it like you're a bouncer in a nightclub. Find an approach that works for you and do it.)

By doing this, you're taking charge of your mental environment and making beautiful upgrades—just as you decluttered your media environment, your home, and your closet, now you're decluttering your mind. This is one of the most powerful things you can do—and the benefits will ripple into every corner of your life.

The BARE Truth

To sum up the big ideas from this chapter, here's a quick metaphor:

Imagine that the thoughts in your mind are guests at a fabulous dinner party. Each thought represents a person you love. These are wonderful people, caring people, people who inspire you to meet—and exceed—your goals. People who make you feel strong and empowered. People who truly love you and want only the best for you. If any uninvited creeps (aka negative thoughts) show up at the doorstep, trying to bust inside and ruin the party, kick these to the curb. They're not welcome.

Here's another way to think about this:

If you were at the playground with your child, and someone came up to your kid and starting yelling horrible things at them—"You're ugly! Worthless! Lazy! Stupid!"—would you just sit there doing nothing? Hell no! You would say, "Hey creep! Back off! Get out of here! Don't you dare talk to my kid like that!" You wouldn't allow that random stranger to harass your child!

Imagine the child is *you*. Just like you would protect a child against abusive words/thoughts/commentary, protect yourself. When cruel thoughts come into your head, take charge.

Your thoughts are not the boss of you. *You* are the boss of you.

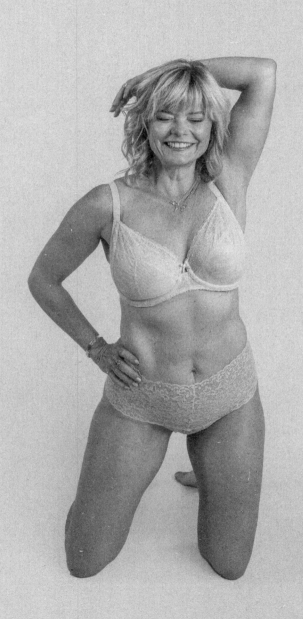

Show Up and Be Seen

*No more hiding. No more slouching down in the
back row. No more waiting on the sidelines. This
is your one, precious life. Show up for it.*

What It Means to Show Up and Be Seen

As a woman, what does it mean to show up and be seen? It means different things for every person. For you, it might mean:

- Wearing a yellow dress that you love instead of that "sensible" navy blue pantsuit that you never liked.
- Being in a family photo instead of ducking away and offering to be the photographer for everybody else.
- Having an important conversation with your partner that you've been putting off.
- Putting together a convincing argument for why you ought to get a raise, and then scheduling a meeting with your boss to talk about it.
- Speaking up when someone makes a racist joke instead of letting it slide.
- Finally starting that podcast you've been thinking about and putting your voice out there in a bigger way.

When I talk about "showing up," I am talking about moving through the world with strength and confidence—letting your words and actions indicate, *I have a voice and I'm using it. I have a body and I'm proud of it. I am not hiding. I am here.*

For a very long time, I wasn't comfortable with showing up and being seen. I avoided it. In doing so, I shrank my power, diluted my opinions, and made my life smaller. I opted out, edited myself out, and sometimes, I was literally . . . *missing.*

Missing from Every Photograph

When I look through scrapbooks and photo albums from when my kids were little, there's a noticeable gap in every photo: me.

There's a four-year period of time where my appearances are very spotty depending on my weight. If I felt heavy, I would refuse to be photographed. Or I would cleverly evade the situation, usually by volunteering to take the photo so I wouldn't have to appear in it. If I felt skinny, then I would sometimes allow myself to be photographed, but even then, I would usually suck in my stomach, tuck myself in the back row, hide half of my body behind my husband, stand behind a table, or hold my kids in front of me to cover my midsection. I had a million and one ways to hide my body from the camera.

But it wasn't just family photos. The way I hid from the camera was a metaphor for the way I hid from my entire life. Every day, in big ways and subtle ways, I was trying to disappear. If someone invited me to attend a party, I would decline because I felt embarrassed about my size. Plus, I hated all my clothes and I had nothing nice to wear. If my husband suggested a tropical beach vacation—forget it. Me? In a bathing suit? On a beach? In *public*? Maybe in a year or two, once I've lost weight. If a neighbor made an insensitive remark or racist joke that really wasn't funny, instead of speaking up to say, "That's not OK," I would bite my tongue. I would keep quiet. I figured, "Nobody wants to hear my opinion." Or, "I don't have the strength to get into an argument right now. I'm just going to keep my mouth shut."

Even after enrolling in a life-coaching certification program—which I felt so excited about—I felt ashamed to tell anyone about it. For a long time, I kept it a secret from everyone except my husband. I figured, "I'm still chubby. Who wants to hire a fat life coach? Nobody."

I hid myself physically. I hid myself professionally. I even hid my spiritual and political beliefs. Technically I was alive—my heart was beating—but I wasn't participating in the action of living. At almost every possible opportunity, I would remove myself or slink off to the sidelines. I was always telling myself, "Later, once I'm skinny. Later. That's when my real life begins."

Looking back, it breaks my heart. All those albums filled with photos of my beautiful kids, my husband. And where am I? Absent. All those years of missed opportunities. All those vacations we could have taken. All those memories we could have shared together. I said "no" to so much joy. And for what? Because my tummy wasn't flat enough?

If there is a God, Goddess, or universal force watching over us, I imagine God was watching me during that time with so much sadness and frustration, thinking, *Susan, I gave you this incredible body. I gave you this beautiful life. This is your one shot to enjoy everything I have given to you. Please, Susan. This is it. Don't waste this.*

Start with One Turtle Step

Clients often ask me, "Susan, how did you stop hiding? How did you start showing up in your life?"

Here's the answer: It didn't happen overnight. There was no crash of thunder and lightning. There was no instant epiphany. It was a slow, gentle process filled with hundreds of tiny turtle steps.

While browsing through my local bookstore, I noticed a book called *Finding Your North Star* by Dr. Martha Beck. Something about the book sang out to me. My intuition said, *You need this book.* It wasn't the type of book that I typically read, but I listened to the zing of excitement inside my body and bought it anyway. That was one turtle step.

Back at home, I ran a bath for myself and slipped inside with my new book. By the third or fourth page, I was sobbing. Martha's writing was exactly what my heart needed. It felt like having a comforting, encouraging conversation with a mentor that I didn't even know I needed. I promised myself I would google Martha's name and learn more about her. That was another turtle step.

The next day, at my computer, I did some googling. I discovered that Martha didn't just write books—she also taught various types of training programs. My body's intuition pinged me again. *Sign up right now! Do one of these programs. Go!* I picked up the phone and made the call.

Within minutes, I was enrolled to attend a personal development class with Martha in Arizona. As luck would have it, there was exactly one spot left. I'd never done anything like this before. But I knew it felt right. After years of hiding, after years of promising myself, *Maybe next year* . . . I was taking decisive action to make something happen *right now.*

No waiting. No postponing. NOW. It felt terrifying, of course. But also incredibly empowering.

Then a few weeks later, there I was: Getting on a plane, lifting into the sky, heading to Arizona to meet Martha. I was going to show up—literally—to meet my new hero. That was a hugely important step.

Each time I listened to my body's intuition. Each time I chose love instead of self-harm. Each time I chose to show up (even if it was in a very small, subtle way) instead of hiding. Each time, I took one more turtle step forward. And with each turtle step forward, my confidence soared. A few months down the road, I noticed myself choosing to show up a lot more frequently, and in all kinds of different ways.

I started to be honest and vocal about my spirituality after years of avoiding the topic: "Actually, I don't go to church anymore. I am spiritual but not religious."

I started to be honest about my political and social values instead of worrying that I might be offending the people around me. I decided that if someone got offended, tough cookies. I'm not going to be a silent woman: "I absolutely think gay and lesbian people should be allowed to get married. Of course. No question."

I started to be honest about what kind of mom I wanted to be. Turtle step by turtle step, my husband and I worked it out, coming up with new plans and family routines that didn't exhaust me. (Or him.) I was able to say aloud, "I love reading to the kids. I love telling stories to them at bedtime. But I hate doing the afternoon carpool. We need to figure out another solution."

Once you stop hiding—once you taste what it feels like to show up and be fully engaged and vocal in your life—it's pretty exhilarating. That doesn't mean it's always easy. Unfortunately, not everyone was thrilled to meet the new me.

Dealing with More Attention: Fans, Supporters, and Haters, Too

Over the past ten years, I have evolved physically, emotionally, and professionally.

I've become more outspoken. I've become extremely clear about my boundaries. I don't allow people to mistreat me or waste my time. I've subtracted toxic relationships from my life (with no apologies). I've become much, much clearer about what I stand for and what I am willing to fight for.

As a life coach, I want to teach other women how to embrace these values today. Life is a precious gift, and the clock is always ticking. This is it. No time to waste. I'm here to help women discover how strong they can be. I'm here to help you become the type of woman who treats her body with excellent, loving care. The type of woman who chooses to love herself, not harm herself. The type of woman who has the energy to meet—and exceed—her goals. The type of woman who doesn't sleepwalk through life, hide from life, or postpone life until "someday later." The type of woman who *shows up.*

As I've evolved, and as I've grown stronger and more self-assured, two things have happened:

I've attracted a passionate, supportive, loving community of friends, allies, clients, and customers from all around the world. Thousands of women who say, "Yaaas, Susan! Preach it!" and who love seeing me express myself to the fullest.

I've also attracted a small—but equally passionate—throng of vitriolic haters. People who see me writing, podcasting, speaking onstage, or posting photos and videos online and who respond with hate mail or even death threats. Bullies who want me to shut up. Bullies who feel threatened by the sight of my body—or the sound of my voice—and who want me to disappear.

Every time I post a photo of myself enjoying my body—leaping into the lake, wearing a bikini, strutting down the street in a slinky outfit—that's when I get an especially huge deluge of hate mail. There's something about seeing a woman who is enjoying her life—and enjoying her body—that sends these haters into a rage vortex.

"You call yourself a feminist? You're an embarrassment."

"What kind of mother posts photos like that online? Slut. I feel bad for your kids."

"You claim to be all about 'women's empowerment,' but how can you say that? You're just taking advantage of desperate women, selling the same old 'weight-loss' B.S. like everyone else."

"Women like you make me sick."

Those are actual messages that I have received via email and on Facebook.

I know. It seems unbelievable. Who says something like that? Who does that? Well, sadly, lots of people do. There's something about the semi-anonymity and virtual distance of the internet that makes it easy for bullies to say all kinds of awful things that they'd probably never say to my face.

I don't like getting hate mail. I don't like feeling attacked or rejected. Nobody does. It's never fun when someone tells you, "You should be ashamed of yourself." (Even if you know that their words are not true, it still stings.)

Obviously, some people do not like the fact that I refuse to hide my body or my opinions. Some people get really, really upset about this. But you know what? Let them be upset. They can rant and rage all they like. They can even send me hate mail if they must. Meanwhile, I'll be right over here, doing my thing, pursuing my dreams, celebrating my body, and enjoying my life.

I spent years hiding from the world—hiding from cameras, hiding from parties, hiding from conversations, hiding from experiences that I really craved—and I refuse to hide anymore. Not for one more second. Haters gonna hate. But I will not stoop to that level. And I won't pretend to be someone I'm not.

As Michelle Obama says, "When they go low, we go high." Damn straight. We go high. And we don't hide.

Coming Out of the Cave

It was spring break and my husband wanted to take the whole family to San Antonio, Texas, for a weekend trip. At this point in my life, I had lost ten out of the thirty-five pounds that I'd been hoping to lose. I was eating much more attentively, doing my Pilates three times a week, walking every day, and learning how to manage my stress levels without diving into the refrigerator for comfort. I was proud of my progress, but I still had a long way to go before I was at my natural/goal weight.

I remember looking into my bedroom mirror, assessing my body. I was undeniably slimmer. I had dropped down a whole clothing size. For the trip to Texas, I decided to dress a little more boldly. I decided to bare my skin just a little bit more than usual. I packed a sleeveless white tank top. At that time in my life, wearing a "sleeveless white tank top" felt like a wild, salacious display of public nudity. It was a big deal for me.

During the trip, we visited a cave and took a fascinating tour through the caverns. We all wore yellow construction hardhats with flashlights strapped to the top. The kids loved it. I held my husband's hand as we toured through the cave, feeling grateful to be there with him, feeling blessed that we could share this experience together, exploring this natural wonder. I mean, how often do you get to descend into the mouth of a cave?

At the end of the tour, as we clambered back up to the surface, the tour guide offered to take a group photo of the entire family. My husband, Scott, enthusiastically accepted. I felt myself cringe.

Even though I'd made so much progress, and even though I'd lost quite a bit of weight, getting my photo taken was still an uncomfortable proposition. I really wanted to duck out. I wanted to invent some type of excuse to avoid it. ("I need a bathroom break! You guys go right on ahead without me!") But I knew that those impulses weren't necessarily healthy or helpful. I knew that was my inner mean girl talking, bullying me, trying to make me feel unworthy and afraid.

I also knew that it was important not to delete myself from my own life. I knew that, one day, my kids would really love to have this photo of mom and dad at the San Antonio caves. I didn't want to steal that away from them.

So, I summoned up my courage. I snuggled close to my husband. I smiled.

Click.

We purchased the photo and took it home.

This is the part of the story where you might be expecting me to say, "… and the photo was GORGEOUS, and I loved it and I never felt critical about my body again! Hooray!"

Nope. That's not how this story goes. Honestly, I hated the cave photo. I thought my arms looked flabby. I thought my smile looked awkward and forced (probably because it was). Looking at the photo triggered a flurry of unhappy emotions. And yet, I was still proud of myself for doing it. I knew that staying in the frame was an important personal milestone. I allowed myself to be photographed. I allowed myself to be seen. It was prickly. It was uncomfortable. It triggered some emotional gunk that I had to deal with and clear away. But I did it. And I can do it again.

When I look at the cave photo today, many years later, I feel very different emotions. I don't feel disgust. I feel compassion for that younger, more anxious version of me. I remember her pain. I remember her sense of longing for a different body, one that felt like home. I feel proud of her for being brave enough to step in front of that camera. Because of her bravery, my family has a precious memento of a very special adventure.

We went to the caves. We had a beautiful time. They took a photo, and I'm in it. I was there.

I chose not to erase myself from the story.

The Secret to Great Photos? Send Love into the Camera

Sometimes, a very special angel comes into your life and you just know you'll never be the same. My friend Chelsea Sanders is one of those people.

I hired Chelsea to take some photos of me for my website. I wanted to look professional—you know, like a life coach that you could trust—but also warm and welcoming. I didn't want to look stiff, awkward, or corporate. No beige blazers allowed. Those days were long gone. I wanted to look like the best possible version of me, like the real me.

I explained all of this to Chelsea, somewhat nervously. I'd never done a professional photo shoot before, and I wasn't sure what to expect. Was she going to make me strut down the street like a supermodel on a runway? Was she going to make me rest my chin on top of my fist and tilt my head subtly to the left, like a high school yearbook photo? Was this whole thing going to be a big waste of time and money?

Like the pro that she is, Chelsea sensed my nervous jitters and was unfazed. She knew exactly what to say to help me relax.

"Look into the camera lens," she told me. "And pretend that you're looking at Scott."

My sweet, amazing husband, Scott. I pictured him in my mind. I felt my shoulders relax, dropping down, falling away from my ears. My smile shifted from forced to genuine. My body language softened. Instead of fretting about how I looked, my attention went in a new direction. I thought about Scott. I thought about love.

Click.

"These are going to be amazing," Chelsea assured me.

A few days later, when Chelsea showed me the finished photos, I was stunned. My eyes sparkled. My face glowed. These photos had personality, energy, warmth. They were alive.

"Oh my God! Oh my God!" I squealed for approximately fifteen minutes straight.

"I told you!" Chelsea said.

After that, I conducted a little experiment. Every time I was being photographed—by myself, by a friend, or by a professional—I would picture someone in my mind, and I would send that person a message of love.

I would picture my two kids and think, "I love you."

I would picture one of my favorite clients and think, "I love you."

I would stare right into my own eyes for a selfie and think, "I love you."

Instantly, all of my photos just looked better. When you're thinking about love, channeling love, transmitting love through your body, it shows.

Not long ago, I shared this discovery with a client of mine. She hired me for weight-loss coaching, and she asked for my advice on posing for photos.

"You always look amazing in photos, Susan," she told me. "But I always feel so awkward."

She explained to me that, in every photo, she's always fidgeting, fussing, sucking in her stomach, or worrying she's going to look fat. Consequently, she always "looks weird," in her words, like she's uncomfortable being there in the shot. And she is.

"Look into the camera and think, 'I love you,'" I told her. "Stop focusing on the size of your body. Place your attention somewhere else. Send a love message through your eyes. Send it to the camera."

She tried this. Now her photos look completely different. She looks relaxed, more confident, like there's pure love beaming directly from her face.

When you send love to the camera, it loves you back.

Danielle's Story
Love Is Not Optional

There's a woman named Danielle Cohen (danielle-cohen.com) who's a friend of a friend of mine. Danielle had her first baby in her early twenties, followed by several more kids.

In one of her online courses for women, she writes: "The pregnancies had created a rippling, crisscross pattern of stretch marks on my stomach. I hated the way it looked."

Danielle is a photographer who specializes in honoring and celebrating women's bodies. Yet, just like so many of her clients, she has sometimes struggled to celebrate her own body—especially her stomach.

"It took many, many years before I became capable of looking at my bare belly—marks, bumps, and all—without feeling painful self-loathing," she says. "Even more years before I could gaze at the middle of my body with love and genuine pleasure. Today, as a woman in my forties going through yet another body transformation, I find my belly quite beautiful yet have had to move on to embracing the new shapes, tones, and forms of other body parts. For years, my gaze would often tend to 'skip' my belly. When I'd look in the mirror, it was above or below. Rarely directly at my stomach."

When you repeatedly refuse to look at (or touch) a particular part of yourself, your body knows. It can feel your disgust and disappointment, just like a small child cowering in the face of a judgmental parent. Danielle knows this and did a lot of work to transmute those feelings into something much truer and more powerful.

With practice, Danielle has learned how to give her stomach the love that it deserves. She likes to rub essential oils into her belly. She's a fan of self-massage. She also uses photography as a way of seeing herself and of documenting and honoring her body and all the amazing things it can do.

"It's not always been easy for me, but I learned how to love you, belly," she writes. "Because you are part of me. The center of me. And loving myself is not optional."

Alex's Story
I Won't Delete Myself

Not long ago, a girlfriend of mine got booked to do a speaking engagement at a gorgeous historic theater. It was a completely packed house with hundreds of people in the audience. She worked hard for weeks leading up to the event and she SLAYED it. The audience exploded into applause. The producers of the show said, "When can we have you back again?" It was a total slam-dunk on every level. She felt so proud.

"Great job! We'll post the video of your performance online in few weeks!" the producers told her.

"Cool!" she said. And she meant it.

But then a few days after the event, my friend found herself glancing in the mirror and wondering, *I wonder if I will look chunky in the video when they post it online? Ugh. Maybe I picked the wrong outfit. That top was a bad idea. I should have worn all black.* For about twenty minutes, my friend considered asking the producers not to post her video online. Ever. (You know. Just in case she looked fat.)

I am happy to report: She came to her senses. She didn't email the producers to make that request. She realized that her mind had temporarily fallen into a fear spiral, and she needed to pull herself out of it. She took some deep breaths. She reminded herself, *I am awesome.* She also reminded herself, *In my talk, I tell a really important personal story. It's a story that thousands of young gay, lesbian, and bisexual people need to hear. It's a story that will help so many people feel less afraid and less alone. If this video doesn't go up, then those people won't get to hear my story. And all because I think I might look fat? Come on. No way, dude. I'm not going to delete myself from the internet like that.*

She wrestled with her fears, and she won. The video went up. Her story went out. She chose to show up—not hide. And she helped countless LGBT kids with her message.

No More Hiding

Ask yourself the following questions:

- How many times in the past year have you strategically cropped and filtered a photo to make yourself look skinnier? (God forbid the internet see your actual arms or butt.)
- How many times have you shied away from some type of public event, party, or experience because you didn't think you'd look thin, young, or hot enough?
- How many times have you tucked yourself into the back row of a photo—or eagerly volunteered to be the photographer to avoid having to be in the picture?
- How many times each week do you catch a glimpse of yourself in the mirror and think some variation of *Ugh, gross*?

I bet your answer to all of those questions is *More times than I would like to admit.*

You're not alone. It's sick and sad, but that's the norm. Most women hate their bodies (a whopping 97 percent of women, according to one study). It's actually rare to find a woman who doesn't. We all need to fight to change this.

The change begins with you, on an individual level: It begins when you actively fight to stop negative thoughts in their tracks. It begins when you put yourself in front of the camera lens, not just behind it. It begins when you choose to show up for your life and allow yourself to be seen.

The next time you hear that ugly voice inside your mind—that voice that says, *Crop that photo! Suck in your stomach! Skip that vacation; you don't deserve it! Get in the back row! Get rid of that video; delete it so no one can see!* I urge you, don't listen to that voice. Don't hit the delete button on yourself. Don't silence yourself. Don't crop out your limbs. Don't hide your story. Don't fade into the background of your life.

You are needed in this world. You have work to do in this lifetime. Step forward to center stage.

I know it's scary. I know you feel shaky and vulnerable, sometimes, to be seen. But you came into this world full of love, curiosity, and delight about your body—and you can get back to that loving place again. I promise you.

Those ugly, destructive voices don't have to rule over you. You can rise above them. You are strong enough.

Repeat after me: *I will not delete myself.*

Bare Yourself to the World

I'll never forget my client who—in her sixties—wore a bikini in public for the very first time. "My stomach had never felt the sunshine before," she told me. I wept.

Another client felt like her voluptuous breasts were a curse. During her teenage years, boys would always stare, often making lewd, inappropriate comments. As she grew older, she discovered clever ways to downplay her shape. She'd wear dark colors and high necklines to draw attention away from her chest. She always dressed extremely modestly—not because she particularly wanted to, but because she felt she had to. It was a protective mechanism. A shield.

One day, during our work together, she decided to do something totally wild and brazen—wear a V-neck top in public. Not a plunging neckline, just a modest V-shape that showed the faintest hint of cleavage. For some women, this type of top would be no big deal, but for her, this was a revolutionary choice.

The experience was totally empowering. Afterward, she told me that it felt like she was reclaiming her body. Like she was sending a message to all those dumb teenage boys who had tormented her in the past: "You can be as stupid as you like, and you can stare all you want, but you do NOT have the power to make me feel bad about myself. I will not cover myself up because of YOU."

It's incredible how a few inches of fabric or skin can symbolize so much: authority, empowerment, discernment, and agency.

Another client went jogging on a warm, sunny day and started to feel a bit warm. In the middle of her jog, in broad daylight, in public, she peeled off her t-shirt and finished her workout wearing just a sports bra on top—something she'd never done before in her entire life. Even though she's not at her goal weight yet, and even though her stomach is a little more jiggly than she'd like it to be, she felt beautiful and strong.

"I did it for all the girls out there who feel less than what they are," she told me, "And I did it for me. Just for me."

As all of these women discovered, it is incredibly powerful to bare yourself to the world. You can bare yourself with a clothing choice—whether it's a bikini, a V-neck top, or a bare midriff. You can also bare yourself with an essay, with a speech, with a bold career choice, with something that has nothing to do with your clothing or physical form.

When you allow people to see you—the real you, uncovered and unmasked—the effects can be life-altering. It's like allowing yourself to be the heroine of your own story instead of a sidekick character. It's like moving from the wings of the stage into the spotlight—right where you belong.

Your Assignment
Take One Selfie Every Day for Seven Days

Documenting yourself on camera can be a powerful way to give your body some love. It's also a powerful way to remind yourself: *I am alive. My life is happening right now. I'm not hiding out. I'm showing up.*

This week, your assignment is to take seven selfies. One selfie per day. You can publicly share your selfie or not.

Day 1: Take a selfie of your feet.

Day 2: Take a selfie of your favorite body part.

Day 3: Take a selfie of your face.

Day 4: Take a #nofilter makeup-free selfie, first thing in the morning.

Day 5: Take a bedtime selfie as you're cozily snuggled in your bed.

Day 6: Take a full-length selfie of yourself. Use a bathroom mirror and capture your reflection. Or use the timer feature on your camera.

Day 7: Take a selfie of your least favorite body part.

With each photo, as you're gazing into the camera, or as you're pointing the camera at a particular part of your body, think the words *I love you.*

When you send a message of love to yourself, you can feel it, and it shows up in your photos. Try it both ways: Take a photo when you're thinking of love and one when you're not, and see the difference for yourself.

Keep showing up. In the days, weeks, and months ahead, continue finding new ways to more actively show up in your life.

Choose an area of your life where you usually hide in the background, and make an effort to show up more honestly and more courageously. Maybe there's a conversation that you really need to have with your spouse, child, client, or boss. Maybe you've been postponing that conversation for too long. Go for it. Show up. Spill it. Maybe there's something else you've been postponing for way too long, such as a trip, event, party, or an experience that you keep promising yourself you'll do someday later when you are skinnier. Challenge yourself to do it now. No more waiting. Maybe you run a blog and you want to start writing about topics that you really care about. Challenge yourself to do that. Show up with your true opinions, your true voice. Then, record whatever you notice about the experience. How does it feel to show up in a different way?

_____

_____

_____

_____

_____

_____

_____

Your "real life" doesn't start later, once your body composition is different. Your real life is happening right now.

The BARE Truth

You have your one body. Your one life. Your one chance to
create memories. Your one chance to experience every variety
of sensory pleasure. To love and be loved. To see what your
body can do. To create your unique ripple effect in the world,
touching lives, leaving other people in better condition than
when you found them.

This is it. Your real life doesn't start later. It's now. It's here.
Show up and be seen.

BARE Q&A

OK, so you're working along through the BARE process, and maybe you're already seeing and feeling some changes (yay!). But you have a few questions. That's totally normal.

Here are some of the most common questions and concerns that clients express to me about the BARE process—including what to do if your weight loss seems to be slowing down or stopping, if your partner doesn't support your new lifestyle, or if you're worried that these positive changes won't last.

Common Questions and Concerns After You've Started the Process

Why is it so hard for me to stay consistent with healthy habits?

If you're struggling to stay consistent, the issue is probably a lack of pleasure.

For example, if you schedule workouts on your calendar but then you never go, maybe you're choosing a workout that doesn't feel pleasurable to you. Switch it up. Try something else.

Or, if you're struggling with mindless snacking when you're not even hungry, consider, "What am I really craving? Am I starving for pleasure?" You might be feeling stressed, bored, or craving entertainment, so you're reaching for food because, hey, food is pleasurable! Try to choose another form of pleasure that's not food-related. When you infuse your life with more pleasure, you won't feel that annoying urge to overeat.

Bottom line: When you create a self-care plan that feels pleasurable, it's much easier to stay consistent with it. You won't have to force it. You'll just *want* to do it!

What if my spouse/partner doesn't want me to change my lifestyle? Sometimes I feel like they're trying to sabotage me!

In an ideal world, your partner would be thrilled to see you eating more attentively, moving your body, speaking your mind, living more courageously, and taking excellent care of yourself. In an ideal world, your partner would support you 100 percent.

In many partnerships, that's exactly what happens, and that's always wonderful to see. But unfortunately, some partners struggle to give that type of support. There are lots of reasons why this can happen. More often than not, though, the root of the issue is that your partner feels *anxious*. Your partner sees you evolving, making all kinds of positive changes, looking and feeling different, and your partner begins to worry. He/she might be thinking:

She's going to leave me.

She's too good for me. I don't deserve her.

She's got all these new priorities—like working out—and there's no time left for me anymore.

Eventually she'll get bored of me and drop me—just like she's clearing out so many other aspects of her old life.

Is your partner being a total silly-pants, worrying like that? Maybe. Maybe not. Only you know that for sure.

As you transform your body and your life, it is entirely possible that you will outgrow your current relationship and decide that it's time to move on. I've witnessed that happen many times for my clients.

It's also entirely possible that you will stay with your current partner for many more happy years, or for the rest of your life.

I've been married to the same wonderful man for twenty-five years. He has seen me gain thirty-five pounds. He has watched me try dozens of destructive diets that ravaged my body and my spirit. He has watched me lose thirty-five pounds in a natural, gradual, healthy manner—as outlined in this book. He has watched me transition from couch potato to avid runner. We've been together through it all. And twenty-five years in, our relationship is stronger than ever.

So, if you and/or your partner are freaking out, thinking that doing the BARE process means "the end of our relationship," just know that doesn't necessarily have to be true. It certainly wasn't true for my husband and me. If we ever split up, it will be for one reason, and one reason only: Because country music superstar Keith Urban finally asks me to marry him. (Just kidding, Scott. You know you're the only one for me.)

My advice: If you sense that your partner is unhappy with the fact that you're doing the BARE process, have a conversation about it. Encourage your partner to voice his/her concerns, and try not to interrupt.

If it feels right, give your partner some love and reassurance. Tell him/her: "I have not stopped loving you. I still love you so much. I am just learning how to give myself lots of love, too. I am learning how to become the type of woman who takes excellent care of herself. I hope you can support me in that. Maybe you could join me? Let's make a meal together/ let's go for a walk together . . ."

With that type of reassurance, your partner might feel differently about the changes you're making.

What if I don't want to eat what the rest of my family is eating?

I remember struggling with this! Back when I was in my "repressed, resentful beige-sweater mom phase," I used to think that family dinner meant me, Scott, and the kids gathering around the table at the exact same time, eating the exact same food, at the exact same pace, and cleaning our plates. Anything other than that was a failure.

You know what? That's B.S. If you want to eat dinner two hours after your husband, because that's when your body feels −2 level hungry and asks for food, great! Do that. If your teenage son wants a pork chop but your body is asking for a big spinach salad, or vice versa, cool! Listen to your body and feed it what it wants. Let your body talk to you. Encourage your family members to roll the same way.

It can feel very satisfying to enjoy a family dinner together, all at the same time, but if that doesn't happen every single night of the week, like clockwork, it's not the end of the world.

In my household, we have dinner all together as a family unit some nights—and other nights we don't. Some nights we all eat the exact same food—and other nights we don't. So far, our family is still functioning and neither of my kids have turned into bank robbers or axe murderers. We're just fine. Your family will be, too.

I feel so much better, but my weight isn't changing. What's the deal?

A few possibilities to consider:

> *Maybe you don't need to lose any more weight.*
>
> It's possible that you have arrived at your natural/ideal weight. Everyone has a natural weight—a size/shape that your body wants to be. This is largely driven by genetics. Your natural weight might be higher or lower than you expect. When you reach your natural weight, you feel healthy and energetic, and your body feels at home. Consider the possibility that maybe . . . you've arrived. (Congratulations!)

> *Maybe you need to be patient.*
>
> When you're going through the BARE process, you're going to lose weight gradually and steadily. But you might not lose the exact same amount of weight every single week. If it seems like the number on the scale isn't moving very much, and it's been one or two weeks, be patient. A few weeks from now, things might look and feel different.

> *Maybe it's time to set the scale aside.*
>
> If you've been obsessing over the number on the scale, maybe it's time to turn your attention elsewhere. Even if you're not losing pounds on the scale, it's possible that you're experiencing other types of positive, noticeable changes.

Maybe your ratio of body fat versus lean muscle is changing. (Muscle weighs more than fat.) Maybe your clothes are fitting more loosely. Maybe you can see a bit of muscle definition when you look in the mirror. Maybe you *feel* different, too—more energized, more productive, more focused, hopeful, and excited about the future. In my opinion, your feelings are your number-one best indicator of progress and success.

I've lost weight, but I'm still not happy with my appearance. Now what?

I remember seeing a woman at my local gym who had the type of body that millions of women would kill for. Tall, slim, toned. She was built like a Victoria's Secret model. There she was in the dressing room, moaning into the mirror, complaining to her friend about her elbow wrinkles. Yes. *Elbow wrinkles.*

You can have the body of a twenty-one-year-old Brazilian supermodel, but if you are unhappy on the inside—if you feel miserable about your career, if you feel trapped in your marriage, or if your mind is littered with a constant stream of toxic thoughts that you haven't dealt with yet—then you will always find something to criticize and pick apart. (Hence the elbow wrinkles.)

I would encourage you to revisit Week 6 of the BARE process, where we discuss how to detox your mind. Do that assignment again. Eavesdrop on your thoughts for one day. Every hour, when your timer goes off, write down what you're thinking. Identify thoughts that exhaust you—thoughts that feel harmful and toxic—and do something to clear those thoughts out of your mind. As you might remember, there's a big list of different approaches that you can try inside the chapter for Week 6.

I would also encourage you to find a new hobby to stimulate your mind. Infuse your life with more fun and pleasure. Volunteer at a dog shelter. Study Italian. Get your scuba diving certification. Learn how to do fancy braids in your hair. When you take steps to make your daily life feel more satisfying, often, that hypercritical voice inside your head fades away. Because you're having way too much fun to worry about something silly like elbow wrinkles. When your life feels deliciously satisfying, you'll feel much more satisfied with your physical appearance, too.

I'm doing the BARE process, but I keep overeating. Why does this keep happening?

You probably know, from personal experience, that when you overeat, it feels crappy. You get sleepy, bloated, cranky, and sad. Your digestive system doesn't work at its best. You gain weight. That's the opposite of what you want. So, have a quick pep talk with yourself and remind yourself: *I am stopping my meal because I am satisfied—and because I want to feel energized later, not sleepy and sick.*

When you feel the urge to overeat, try telling yourself this: *I could eat more food right now. But I choose not to. Because I want to feel good now/later/tomorrow.*

As always, it comes back to this question: "What would feel like love?" Continuing to eat (when you're already full) is not a very loving thing to do to your body. So don't do it. Choose love.

If that's not helping, try to bring yourself into a curious frame of mind. Put on your detective hat. If you're continually overeating, there's obviously a reason for that. Try to get to the source of what's going on.

Here are some things to look at:

Are you starving or depriving yourself for most of the day?

Whether consciously or unconsciously, you might be undereating during most of the day, leading to intense hunger and cravings later on.

Maybe you oversleep and you skip breakfast. Then you're racing around and you don't set aside enough time for a satisfying lunch. Then it's dinnertime and you're so hungry, you could practically eat a chunk of cement. Your body is panicking, urging you to eat, eat, eat. Then you wind up overdoing it and you feel uncomfortably stuffed.

This is a common pattern for so many people. The solution is very simple: Eat at regular intervals throughout your day. Rely on your body's natural hunger signals to guide you.

Remember the hunger scale that we discussed during Week 3 of the BARE process? Try to eat something before you hit –3 on the hunger scale. Try to stop eating before you reach +3 on the fullness side of the scale. Do your best to stay between –2 and +2 as often as possible. If you do that, you'll be fueling your body the way it wants to be fueled, and the urge to overeat won't haunt you very often.

Are you tired?

Millions of Americans are chronically sleep deprived. If you don't get enough sleep, your body suffers in myriad ways. For one thing, your cortisol levels shoot up. Cortisol is a "stress hormone" that often leads to intense cravings, particularly sugar cravings. Make sleep a top priority, and you'll notice that the urge to overeat feels less intense.

Are you committed to the idea that you are a "food addict"?

I've had clients say to me, "I can't stop overeating because I am a food addict. It's a mental illness. It's not something that I can control."

Food addiction is a real condition. I'm not denying that. But if you've decided that you are powerless in the face of your addiction, that's not a very productive mind-set.

To transform your life, and to stop bingeing, you have to decide that you are *powerful*, not powerless. If you've already predecided that change is impossible, then . . . change is impossible.

Hire a therapist or a life coach if you feel like you're struggling to change your mind-set on your own. Don't be ashamed if you need to seek professional help. Every Olympic athlete has a coach. Every presidential candidate has a speechwriter. Every CEO has a business mentor. We all need someone to help us tap into our strength and show us what's possible. To create massive change in the world, or in your own life, sometimes it takes a village.

Is there something you are trying to avoid?

Overeating is often driven by a desire to avoid . . . *something.* Is there something you are trying to avoid thinking about, avoid doing, avoid discussing, or avoid feeling?

If you've got a mountain of mind-numbing paperwork sitting in front of you, and you really don't want to do it, that pint of Ben & Jerry's might seem like a really good distraction.

If you're enrolled in a graduate school program, and you've realized that it's not the right program for you, but you're ashamed to admit that to your professors (or your parents), well then hello, Doritos! You might dive headfirst into a jumbo-sized bag of chips as a way of postponing the tough decisions that you know you need to make.

Try to be completely honest with yourself. Make a list of everything that you're trying to avoid or postpone. Then, instead of eating to stuff down your feelings, make the more courageous choice: *Do the one thing that you've been avoiding the most.*

OMG. I know. It's the most annoying advice, right? You probably want to toss this book across the room. But trust me. Do it. Get it over with. Because it's eating you up inside. You'll feel so much better afterward, and the urge to overeat will finally leave you alone.

How can I say "I love my body" and want to lose weight at the same time? Is that even possible? Am I a hypocrite?

No, you're not a hypocrite. Consider this:

Can you love your country AND also want to change your country (gun law reform, better mental health care programs, higher pay for teachers)? Yes.

Can you love your marriage AND also want to change certain aspects of your marriage (more date nights, more sex, less squabbling about chores)? Yes.

Can you love your body AND also want to change your body (new hair color, new tattoo, gain weight, lose weight, whatever)? Yes.

You can love something deeply AND feel excited to change that same thing.

Human beings are capable of holding more than one feeling/desire at the same time. We are MAGICAL like that.

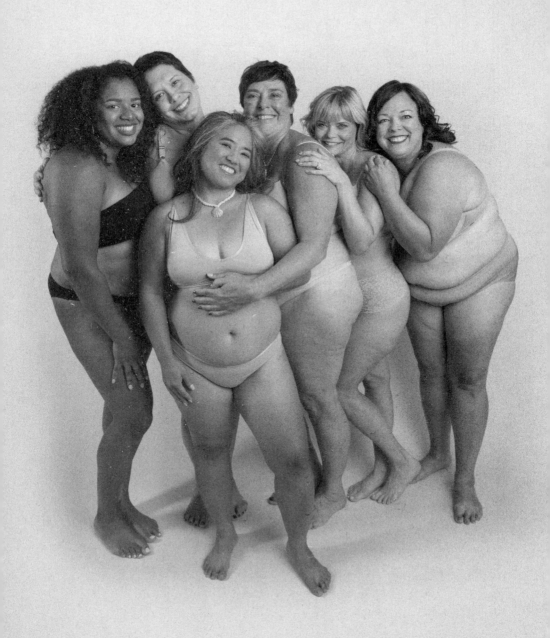

BARE Forever

When I teach the BARE process, I typically break it down into a seven-week sequence. Each week, as you've just seen, there's a new topic and a new assignment to complete. But that doesn't mean that your BARE experience is "over" at the end of the seventh week.

BARE isn't a seven-week diet that you suffer through, begrudgingly, until it's finally over. It's the opposite of that. It's not a diet. It's not a temporary fix. It's a permanent, lifelong promise that you make to yourself.

In this section, we'll talk about how to avoid slipping back into old patterns, and how to keep the BARE principles alive in your life for the long haul.

Backsliding into Old Habits—and How to Avoid This

I've seen clients backslide into old, unhealthy habits because of an *I deserve it!* mind-set. I can relate. Sometimes my thoughts start going there, too.

Like this one time, I was reaching the end of a chaotic, high-tension week. The type of week where everything that could possibly go haywire did: Ryan was having more high school drama. The beagle dashed out the door and refused to come home. Someone forgot to feed the ferret (yes, we have a ferret who lives in our basement—don't ask). My husband was pouting because I needed to fly out of town for a work trip, again, and he missed me and wanted me to stay home. My online shopping cart broke, and several thousand dollars that were supposed to be deposited into my bank account didn't land there. Oh, and I discovered that a blogger had been plagiarizing my work and passing it off as her own—literally reposting my personal life stories from *my* blog onto *her* blog. I felt so violated. This week was absolute insanity.

When Friday afternoon rolled around, I found myself eyeing a bag of spicy Doritos. I rarely eat Doritos anymore, but, for some reason, in that moment, they looked very appealing. As you know by now, there's nothing wrong with eating junk food on occasion—in moderation—so I dove in. I didn't eat an obscene number of chips. Maybe twenty chips in total. They didn't taste quite as amazing as I thought they would, but . . . meh. I ate them anyway.

Licking the neon orange powder off my fingertips, I proudly thought, *This is my special treat. I deserve this.* The past week had been so chaotic. These Doritos were my big reward.

Later that night, I woke up flushed with heat and with a burning pain in my chest. Ugh. Gross. Acid reflux. I'd been telling myself, *This is my special treat* and *This is my big reward for surviving such a tough week.* But that's a ludicrous line of thinking. My "special treat" is excruciating heartburn? My "big reward" is waking up in the middle of the night feeling awful? That's not much of a "treat."

Next time, I promised myself. *I'll choose a different type of reward.*

Instead of munching on food that doesn't make you feel good, and saying, "I deserve this," try asking yourself: *What do I really deserve? What would energize me? What would help me feel good an hour from now? Tomorrow morning?*

Those types of questions can help steer you toward more loving, respectful choices.

More Sneaky, Unhelpful Thoughts—and What to Do When They Arise

While cruising in my car with a girlfriend of mine, the topic of conversation turned to alcohol. Specifically: fancy cocktails.

"I don't drink very much compared to lots of people I know," she told me. "I rarely have more than one drink per day. But I've noticed that lately, I have one drink EVERY SINGLE DAY. It's become a nightly ritual. After finishing my work for the day, my boyfriend and I mix up some cocktails with lots of fancy ingredients, like fresh ginger and mint. We tell ourselves, 'Yay! We made it through the day! We got our work done! It's time to relax and celebrate. I deserve it.'"

There's that phrase again: *I deserve it.*

It's amazing how your mind can trick you into thinking you "deserve" something, and how that thought can become twisted into a rationale for overindulging and, ultimately, feeling crappy.

Another round of cocktails? *Sure, I deserve it!*

Slice of cake? *Yes! I deserve it!*

Another slice? *Why not, it's Friday!*

Same thing again tomorrow? *Totally! I deserve it.*

And so on. And so on. It's a seductive line of thinking that so many women fall into. That's why it's so important to continually check in with yourself to ask, *What do I really deserve?* and *What's going to help me feel great later today?*

I deserve it isn't the only thought that trips people up—there are many, many others. I call these types of thoughts "repeat offenders" because they're incredibly common, and often very repetitive. And because they're very sneaky and malicious gateways for destructive behavior. Let's take a look at what you can do—and say—when these types of thoughts clamor into your mind:

Thought: *I'm on vacation!*
Translation: *I can overindulge.*

You're on vacation? Awesome! Taking a vacation is all about resting, recharging, and experiencing pleasure. Is stuffing yourself to the point of discomfort going to feel restful, restorative, and pleasurable? Uh, probably not.

Thought: *But it's the weekend!*
Translation: *I'm going to drink an entire bottle of wine and eat way past the point of fullness.*

Do you want to spend your weekend out of commission feeling bloated and sluggish? Didn't think so. Try to stop eating when you reach +1 or +2 on the hunger scale and your weekend will be a lot more fun and full of energy.

Thought: *Life is short!*
Translation: *I should eat three different desserts and lick the plate clean.*

It sure is. Life doesn't come with any guarantees. You could die seventy years from now . . . or seven hours from now in a tragic car crash. (Let's hope not.) Since life is so brief, don't you want to feel energetic, healthy, confident, and strong, so that you can enjoy it to the fullest? (I would hope so.)

Thought:	*I'll never be at this legendary restaurant again! This is my one and only chance to try their world-famous cheesecake.*
Translation:	*I'm going to eat an obscene amount of cheesecake because I can't have it later.*

Life is meant to be savored—and yes, that includes savoring delicious food. If you're really excited to try something, then try it! Have a few bites, eat attentively and slowly, and maximize every ounce of pleasure from the experience. Then stop when your body tells you, *That's enough.* Honor that.

By doing this, you'll be able to walk away from that legendary restaurant with a positive memory instead of a negative one. Looking back, you'll be able to say, "I had such a great time at that restaurant!" instead of, "I ate until I felt sick and now I can't even think of that cheesecake without getting a little queasy."

Thought:	*Let's not let it go to waste.*
Translation:	*I intend to eat every scrap of this food because each crumb represents money and effort I've spent.*

Dumping unused food into the garbage is never fun. It can feel wasteful, for sure. But you have plenty of options: You can donate food to people who need it. You can compost it. You can freeze it/save it. You can make an effort to cook less next time.

But gobbling down every last crumb just so you're not "wasting" it is not the best choice. If you wind up flopped on the couch, bloated and uncomfortable, too full to even move, then you're "wasting" a big part of your day all because you didn't want to waste food.

How do you want to feel thirty minutes from now? Or an hour from now? Satisfied? Or sick and sluggish? Eat accordingly.

Thought: *This is a really stressful time for me.*
Translation: *I'm allowed to eat excessively and skip exercise sessions.*

If you're going through a really stressful time, then your body needs *more* love, not less. This is the time to ramp up your self-care, not delete it. By eating attentively, and exercising with love, you'll bring down your cortisol (stress hormone) levels, and you'll be better equipped to deal with everything that's stressing you out.

Give your body a gift—the gift of loving, attentive care—instead of giving your body even more stress and discomfort.

Thought: *Girls' night out! We're celebrating!*
Translation: *Let's get trashed!*

Hooray! Celebrate life by making choices that make you feel *more alive*. Choices that energize you. Not choices that make you feel stuffed, sluggish, or wretchedly hungover. Puking into a toilet, feeling constipated, or gaining weight from excessive partying is not exactly a "celebration of life," is it?

If you notice any of those "repeat offender" thoughts creeping into your mind as you go about your daily life, interrupt yourself. Talk back. Consider what you really deserve and how you really want to feel. Make choices that carry you closer toward those feelings, not farther away.

What Would You Say to a Friend?

Many people assume that because I lost thirty-five pounds, and because I've kept off that weight for ten years, that I no longer feel the urge to overeat or mindlessly snack. But that's not true.

I don't feel the urge to overeat as often as I used to—using the BARE process helps to reduce those types of urges tremendously—but I still feel the urge occasionally.

Probably once or twice a week, on average, I'll catch myself in the midst of a moment of thinking, *I might as well polish off the rest of the bag . . .* or *How about another glass of Prosecco? I deserve it.* The difference is that, now, I know how to manage those feelings when they bubble up, and I know how to coach myself away from a decision that I might regret later.

Have you ever received a phone call from a friend who was really distressed? Maybe she was going through a terrible breakup, and she was thinking about slashing her ex's tires, or chopping off all of her hair, or drinking an entire bottle of whiskey, or some other poor decision that she'll regret later.

What would you say to your friend? You'd probably try to comfort her, right? You'd try to calm her down. Try to reason with her. You'd probably say to her: "Hey, sweetheart, I know you're in pain right now, and that is totally understandable. But don't go slash his tires, OK? That's not a productive way to deal with everything you're feeling. You're just going to make a bad situation even worse. And you might regret it later." You would try to talk your friend off the ledge, so to speak.

You can talk to yourself in the exact same way when you're about to make a bad decision for your well-being.

When you're reaching into the freezer, feeling the urge to polish off two or three ice cream sandwiches, you can interrupt yourself in the midst of that moment. You can coach yourself off the ledge, just like you're talking to a good friend. You can even speak to yourself aloud, "Hey, whoa. I know you're feeling sad/irritated/lonely/anxious/bored right now, and you're totally allowed to feel that way. But eating three ice cream sandwiches is not the answer. Think about how you want to feel an hour from now. Think about how you want to feel when you wake up tomorrow morning. You want to feel healthy, strong, and energetic, right? Would eating three ice cream sandwiches help you to feel that way? Probably not. So back up. Close the door. Find something else to do. Choose love."

This is such a simple, obvious-sounding concept—*talk to yourself like a good friend*—but it's amazing how effective it can be.

How Do You Want to Feel in Your Life?

In her best-selling book, *The Desire Map*, Danielle LaPorte poses the question: "How do you want to feel in your life?"

She invites you to mull it over, talk it out with a friend, or do some journaling to come up with specific words to describe your "Core Desired Feelings" (aka CDFs, the primary feelings that you want to feel as you move through your everyday life). Maybe you want to feel sexy, affluent, and electric. Or maybe you want to feel generous, prolific, and vivacious. Or focused, athletic, and purposeful. You get the idea.

After you've written down your Core Desired Feelings, Danielle invites you to "act the way you want to feel." One exercise that she recommends is to make a list of five to ten different experiences that will help to generate the feelings you most want.

If I want to feel "powerful," I could generate that feeling today by doing the following:

- Lifting weights at the gym. ("I am so strong!")
- Spending two hours working on creating materials for my new coaching program. ("I'm a powerful entrepreneur who gets things done!")
- Listening to my body attentively, fueling myself when I'm hungry, and stopping before I get too full. ("I feel nourished and energized and ready to take charge, not sleepy and sluggish.")

If there's a feeling that you desire, you don't have to passively wait for someone to give you that feeling. That's not how it works. You can generate that feeling for yourself, today, by making specific choices that carry you closer to that feeling.

This is another one of those simple, obvious-sounding (yet totally life-changing) practices that you can integrate into your daily life. "Do what it takes," Danielle says, "to feel the way you want to feel."

Fiercely Protect Your Health

I used to have very flimsy boundaries. I didn't think I was allowed to say "Nope!" to anyone—especially not to people in my inner circle, like my husband and my kids. If my daughter, Cora, asked me to drive her to the art store to get supplies for a school project, I'd drop whatever I was doing like a hot potato and get the car revving. If my son, Ryan, needed to ask a question, he'd barge into my home office and start chattering away. It didn't matter if I was on the phone with a potential client, or in the middle of writing a newsletter, or doing my monthly accounting. I'd hop up and help out.

I felt the same way with my clients. When I started my coaching practice—before I learned how to set clear work boundaries—I gave my clients full access to my life around the clock. If a client emailed on a Saturday at 11 PM at night with a concern, I would email back ASAP.

I'm not blaming my kids—or my clients—for behaving this way. It wasn't their fault. It was mine. Because I taught them that it was OK.

Through my daily actions, I sent them a message, and that message was: "It's OK to ask me for anything, anytime, night or day, and I will always jump to serve you instantly." I carried on like this for years, and you know what? It was exhausting.

When you don't set boundaries, it begins to feel like energy is leaking out of your body. It's tedious and tiring. You feel resentful and bitter. The urge to mindlessly snack/overeat/binge-eat can overwhelm you. You wonder why people are constantly taking advantage of your kindness and generosity. Why? Well, because they think it's OK. Because you've never indicated otherwise. It's up to you to set them straight.

Gradually, I began to understand that it was time to re-educate the people around me. I needed to set boundaries—and consistently enforce them—or my physical and mental health was going to continue to suffer.

I had to teach my kids, "When mom's office door is closed, that means NO disruption."

I had to teach my clients, "We can speak on the phone at our appointed time. But I'm not available for spontaneous phone calls or SOS email conversations. That's not the service that I provide."

I had to teach my (highly extroverted) husband, "I am not going out to parties, happy hours, and fund-raisers every single night of the week. It exhausts me. I'll go with you occasionally, but not every time."

Not everyone responded favorably to these new boundaries. People tried to "test" me, to see just how serious I was. My son Ryan, in particular. One night, I remember telling him,

"I'm going jogging tomorrow morning really early, before I take you to school. Which means I'm not going to wake you up or nag you to get out of bed. You're old enough to do that on your own. It's your responsibility to get up, get dressed, and get ready for school. I expect you to be ready to get into the car as soon as I get back from my jog."

He didn't believe me. When I got back from my jog, he was still wearing his pajamas.

"I guess you're going to school in your pajamas," I told him. His jaw hit the floor.

Oh yeah. Mom is not joking around. He didn't test that particular boundary again.

If you hold firm to your boundaries, and refuse to haggle, negotiate, or buckle under pressure, people get the message pretty quickly. You're not a woman to be trifled with. When you say it, you mean it.

Why? Because You Matter

When I encourage my clients to set clear boundaries and fiercely protect their health, they often express resistance.

"I don't want people to think I'm a bitch," some women tell me.

You're not a "bitch." And you're not being stuck up, selfish, or unreasonable either. What you're doing is reminding your-self—and others—that *your life actually matters*. If something is stealing your time, energy, health, sanity, or money . . . if it's harmful . . . if it's exhausting . . . if it's unproductive . . . if it's disempowering . . . then it's got to change.

You simply can't allow that to remain in your life. If you do, that's like saying: "I'm worthless. My life doesn't really matter. My time isn't really that valuable. Go ahead: Suck me dry. Who cares?"

No. Absolutely not. Your life matters. Your health matters.

If believing *my life matters* leads to someone calling you a "bitch," well then, crank up "Work Bitch" by Britney Spears to maximum volume and dance the night away. Consider it a compliment.

You're Becoming *Unstoppable*

My client Natasha recently went through the BARE process. She's a former competitive athlete. For most of her life, she has hated her body. Criticism from abusive coaches weakened her self-esteem and left her feeling like her body was never good enough. The negativity inside her mind was like a lead blanket, weighing her down, impeding her success in every realm of life.

About halfway through the seven-week BARE process, Natasha confessed to me, "I have a secret." I could hear a bit of mischief in her voice.

"What??" I asked. (I love juicy secrets.)

"I've always dreamed about writing a sexy romance novel," she told me. "And I finally feel like I have the energy to do it."

A few months later, Natasha's first novel was finished. She has written three books to date. Something she never thought she was capable of doing.

This woman has always been a high achiever—she's a decorated athlete—but now, it's like she has ascended into a totally different stratosphere of creativity and productivity. The woman is unstoppable.

Now that she's not obsessively tracking her meals (measuring scoops of oatmeal to tabulate every calorie), now that she has cleaned up her environment, and now that she's not talking to herself so cruelly and violently—everything feels different.

She has room in her life, now, to bloom in entirely new directions. Room to pursue her quiet dreams and secret passions. Room to pursue the life that she honestly wants.

You'll experience this type of miracle, too. Like Natasha, you're becoming unstoppable. So much time. So much energy. So much power. Freed up. Liberated. Ready to be channeled into new directions. Ready to be harnessed so that you can do the creative, meaningful work that is calling to you.

Can you imagine what would happen if every woman on the planet could reclaim her power in this way? Can you imagine the symphonies that would be composed, the businesses that would be launched, the inventions that would be patented, the board rooms, companies, and presidential offices that would be flooded with women, ready to take command?

We can create this new world together. It starts on an individual level. It starts with you—with the choices you make about how to spend the hours, days, and years of your life.

Take the BARE Pledge

Right now, I want you to make a promise to yourself—a pledge to take excellent care of yourself, forever and always. You can do it aloud or do it in writing. You can even sign it to make it extra official, like a binding legal agreement. You can phrase your BARE pledge however you want. Here are a few phrases that you might like to use:

I promise to take loving, attentive care of my body because it's the only one I've got.

I promise to continually strip away messages, relationships, obligations, possessions, and thoughts that weigh me down, disempower me, and exhaust me.

I promise not to postpone beautiful experiences that I crave, putting them off until my body has changed.

I promise to always keep learning how to love myself, and how to take care of myself, because there's always room to show up even stronger, always room for more growth.

Love,

[Your Name Here]

Some days, it might feel easy to uphold this pledge. Other days, less so. Do the best you can, every day, knowing that perfection never exists. Keep moving in the direction of love.

You Were Born for Big Things

You were born to create memories. To experience life to the fullest. To create new life, if you choose to. To attempt gutsy projects and make equally gutsy mistakes. To fall in love and discover that, despite piercing heartache, you still have more love to give.

You were born to harness your power and potential and use it to *do something*—whether it's launching your own business, or raising beautiful kids, or designing tiny outfits for tiny dogs, or hosting a hysterical podcast, or running for PTA president or president of the United States.

You were born to do something that matters. Born to create a positive ripple in the world and to leave your mark. (It doesn't have to be a Beyoncé-sized mark, necessarily. It just has to feel authentic and meaningful for you.)

So much power and potential, captured inside your gorgeous, womanly shape.

Don't give your power away. Harness it.

Don't waste your time. Seize it.

Don't ravage your body with violent thoughts and habits. Choose love.

In this moment, you can choose to become the type of woman who takes excellent care of herself. Who believes, *My health matters. My voice matters. My life matters.*

This is not a choice that you need to mull over for the next twenty, thirty, or forty years. This is a choice that you can make right now, a choice that you can keep making every day that you live.

A permanent promise to yourself. With all of my heart: I hope you will make that promise.

> You only get one body. Give it love.
> You only get one life. Make it count.

Join the online community

Inspiration. Sisterhood. Personalized coaching. Life-changing transformation.

If you're inspired by the guidance in this book—and you'd like to connect with other women who are working through the BARE process—you might want to check out the BARE Daily online community.

With a BARE Daily membership, you'll be guided through the seven-week BARE process in a fun, uplifting, and personalized way.

You'll receive one-on-one coaching sessions with a certified BARE coach, where you can ask anything on your mind, share any challenges that are coming up for you, and find realistic solutions to keep you on track.

You'll meet amazing women from around the world who are committed to transforming their bodies in a healthy, empowering manner.

You'll complete weekly assignments to upgrade your environment, eating habits, clothing collection, and more—but instead of working alone, you'll have an entire community cheering you on.

Action + sisterhood + accountability = transformation on every level.

Be part of the BARE movement. Get your BARE Daily membership here: letsgetbare.com.

Become a certified BARE coach

Do you work as a counselor, therapist, life coach, yoga teacher, fitness trainer—any kind of profession related to women's empowerment, health, wellness, weight loss, self-esteem, or body image?

Would you like to add a new credential to your toolkit—and learn new processes to help your clients?

Do you like the idea of leading BARE classes, seminars, or retreats, or incorporating the BARE process into the teaching/coaching work you already do?

Consider becoming a certified BARE coach. Training sessions happen every year. Visit letsgetbare.com for more info.

BARE RESEARCH

A list of studies and articles that were mentioned in this book

Dreisbach, Shaun. "Shocking Body-Image News: 97% of Women Will Be Cruel to Their Bodies Today." *Glamour*, 2 Feb. 2011. http://glamour.com/health-fitness/2011/02/shocking-body-image-news-97-percent-of-women-will-be-cruel-to-their-bodies-today

Frohlich, Thomas C., Alexander Kent, and Mark Lieberman. "The Healthiest Countries in the World." *USA Today*, 3 Apr. 2015.

Gummow, Jodie. "The 12 Most Sexually Satisfied Countries in the World." *Salon*, 19 Feb. 2014. http://salon.com/2014/02/19/the_12_most_sexually_satisfied_countries_in_the_world_partner/

"Lack of Exercise as 'Deadly' as Smoking." *NHS*, 18 July 2012.

Roberts, Christine. "Most 10 Year-Olds Have Been on a Diet: Study; 53 Percent of 13-Year-Old Girls Have Issues with How Their Bodies Look." *New York Daily News*, 3 July 2012. http://nydailynews.com/news/national/diets-obsess-tweens-study-article-1.1106653

Sifferlin, Alexandra. "The Weight Loss Trap: Why Your Diet Isn't Working." *Time*, 25 May 2017. http://time.com/magazine/us/4793878/june-5th-2017-vol-189-no-21-u-s/

Wolpert, Stuart. "Dieting Does Not Work, UCLA Researchers Report." *UCLA Newsroom*, 3 Apr. 2007. http://newsroom.ucla.edu/releases/Dieting-Does-Not-Work-UCLA-Researchers-7832

Books, blogs, podcasts, and documentaries to inspire you

The BARE Podcast

Yes, there's a podcast! Find it on iTunes and on my website: shyatt.com. It's got Q&A, true stories, and interviews with inspiring women.

Embrace

A 2016 documentary film about why poor body image has become a global epidemic—and what women can do to fight back.

The Body Is Not an Apology: The Power of Radical Self-Love by Sonya Renee Taylor

An absolute must-read that challenges body shame and helps us heal with radical self-love.

Shrill: Notes from a Loud Woman by Lindy West

A powerful memoir that deals with many topics, including our culture's obsession with thinness. Soon to be adapted by Aidy Bryant into a Hulu television series.

Stop Fighting Food (isabelfoxenduke.com) by Isabel Foxen Duke

An amazing blog with videos to help you heal your relationship with food.

Body Positive Power: How to Stop Dieting, Make Peace with Your Body and Live by Megan Jayne Crabbe

A powerful read by one the brightest lights online.

The Beauty Myth: How Images of Beauty Are Used Against Women by Naomi Wolf

The best-selling classic that everyone should read.

Food Psych Podcast (christyharrison.com/foodpsych) by Christy Harrison

A helpful blog and podcast by an anti-diet dietician focused on helping people make peace with food.

Health at Every Size: The Surprising Truth About Your Weight by Linda Bacon

An honest look at the truth about health and dieting.

Intuitive Eating: A Revolutionary Program That Works by Evelyn Tribole and Elyse Resch

An eye-opening book for anyone who wants to gain peace with food and get off the dieting roller coaster.

Ifd_bodies (instagram.com/ifd_bodies)
An Instagram account curated by Isabel Foxen Duke that celebrates diversity in body shapes and sizes.

An Epidemic of Beauty Sickness (singjupost.com/an-epidemic -of-beauty-sickness-by-renee-engeln-at-tedxuconn-2013 -full-transcript) by Renee Engeln
A 2013 TEDx Talk on the messages about beauty that girls grow up hearing.

"Let's Talk About Thin Privilege" by Melissa A. Fabello
A 2013 article published in *Everyday Feminism* magazine about thin privilege and "fatphobia."

Things No One Will Tell Fat Girls: A Handbook for Unapologetic Living by Jes Baker
A powerful handbook for fighting fat prejudice and living without shame for those of all ages and sizes.

Fearless Rebelle Radio (summerinnanen.com/blog) by Summer Innanen
A blog and podcast about body image and anti-dieting.

Virgie Tovar (virgietovar.com)
A blog by an expert and lecturer on fat discrimination and body image.

Gratitude

Developing the BARE process—and creating this book—required a village of colleagues, coaches, editors, proofreaders, designers, publishing-industry experts, and so many other friends and supporters.

I'd like to say "thank you" to . . .

Scott Hyatt: My "Silver Fox," who has always been my biggest supporter. (He also had vivid dreams about me sitting on Oprah's couch with this book. #CallMeOprah) Thank you for never letting me quit.

Cora Hyatt: My eighteen-year-old daughter, who teaches me how to be a fierce woman every day. Thank you for being you. You make me so proud to do what I do.

Ryan Hyatt: I actually think my future book, *Raising Ryan*, will be a best seller! No, son, you aren't getting any royalties. Twenty years old and the reason I became a coach. What if you had just behaved in school and I was still selling real estate? #slidingdoors

Brooke Castillo: Brooke was one of my first mentors and helped me turn my attention from external rewards (food) and tune in to my body. Brooke, thank you for years of love and guidance.

Alexandra Franzen: Alex is my writing coach and dear friend. Without Alex, this book might never have happened. Thank you for coming to the lake for a week to help me start this thing.

Frances Cadora: My BFF and running partner. I love you, Frannie Pants!

Larissa Zozula: My right hand and the glue that keeps my biz together. Thank you for helping me every single day.

Katie Kotchman: My agent, who wouldn't let me self-publish. THANK YOU for taking a chance on me and BARE. You are first class.

Maria Teresa Hart: My editor, who made me negotiate for curse words. Because of Maria, dear reader, you were saved from most of my usual language. Thank you for helping make BARE the best it could be.

BenBella Books: Thank you for preserving the spirit and mission of BARE. And, for taking a chance on your next best seller.

Thank you for believing in this work, and for believing in me.

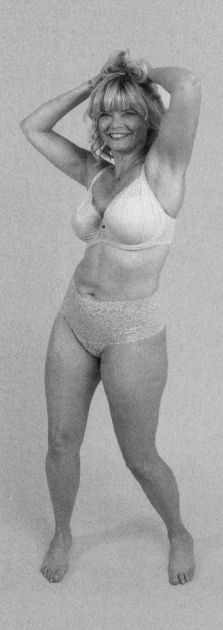

About the Author

SUSAN HYATT is a Master Certified Life and Business Coach based in Evansville, Indiana.

She has been featured on national TV and in magazines like *O: The Oprah Magazine, Cosmopolitan, Seventeen,* and *Woman's World.* In 2017, she was a finalist for the ATHENA Leadership Award, an award recognizing leadership in the field of women's empowerment.

She lives in a house with two dogs, two cats, one ferret, and one Silver Fox (aka her husband, Scott), and has two kids who frequently yell "OMG, sooo embarrassing, Mooom!" when Susan says "Eyebrows on fleek!" or attempts to twerk. Which happens often.

When Susan's not coaching, writing, podcasting, or lighting up Facebook with her impassioned rant of the day, you can find her swinging kettlebells at the gym or lacing up her sneakers for a 5 AM run.

Learn more about Susan—and find tons of free worksheets, training webinars, and motivational pep talks—at shyatt.com and letsgetbare.com.